HOMEO-PATHIC
Medicine Today

Other Keats Books on Homeopathy

HOMEO-PATHIC
Medicine Today

Trevor M. Cook

Keats Publishing, Inc.. New Canaan, Connecticut

Homeopathic Medicine Today is not intended as medical advice. Its intent is purely informational and educational. Please consult a health professional should the need for one be indicated.

HOMEOPATHIC MEDICINE TODAY

Copyright © 1989 by Trevor M. Cook

All Rights Reserved

Library of Congress Cataloging-in-Publication Data

Cook, Trevor M. (Trevor Morgan)
  Homeopathic medicine today.

  Bibliography: p.
  Includes index.
  1. Homeopathy. I. Title. [DNLM: 1. Homeopathy.
WB 930 C77lh]
RX71.C66 1989   615.5'32   88-32837
ISBN 0-87983-473-0

Printed in the United States of America

Keats Publishing, Inc.
27 Pine Street (Box 876)
New Canaan, Connecticut 06840

DEDICATED TO MY MOTHER,
MURIEL COOK

ACKNOWLEDGMENTS

I wish to record my gratitude to all those people who have helped me or inspired me in the writing of this book.

To my daughter, Melodie, for typing the manuscript and to my daughter, Alyson, for their encouragement.

To Jason Adamson, for preparing the diagrams.

To Dr. Christopher Kelsey, for reading and advising me on the manuscript.

To Dr. F. Fuller Royal, Director of the Nevada Clinic, for his assistance with the references to electrodiagnosis and for his friendship.

To my lifelong friends, Garth and Mary Young, and Frank and Doreen Goodman, for their support and encouragement.

To Ann Kingcome for her encouragement.

To Dr. Max Tetau, Medical Director, Dolisos, France, for his inspiration and useful comments on part of the manuscript.

To Muriel Cook, to whom this book is dedicated, and my brother, Charles.

To all my homeopathic friends and associates, worldwide, particularly in the United States, Great Britain and France, whose teachings, example and many acts of kindness have made my involvement in homeopathy so rewarding.

PREFACE

I have presented the subject matter in a logical sequence—history, principles of homeopathy, the sources and preparation of the medicines, prescribing, treatments and the future of homeopathy. I have also included a list of the medicines and some useful information. It is written in a style which I hope will be readily understandable, even to the informed lay reader.

In writing this book I have aimed not to present homeopathy as monolithic, but as a modern, dynamic, vibrant and flexible therapy which is alert to current medical and scientific developments. New advances must be integrated into homeopathy if it is to continue to be an intrinsic part of the whole fabric of medicine. I would stress, however, that this view is not incompatible with the fundamental Hahnemann precepts. The Law of Similars must remain the foundation of homeopathy, now and in the future. I make no excuses, therefore, for quoting Hahnemann at every opportunity.

I have classified homeopathic medicines according to the manner in which they are prescribed, as well as by their sources. The different approaches to treatment are not presented as alternatives, but rather as the whole spectrum of homeopathic practices from which a particular course may be chosen according to the needs of the patient. As with any discipline, homeopathy has its areas of contention, but I have tried not to be too dogmatic, and have left it to the reader to draw his or her own conclusions in these areas.

It is my belief that one of the fundamental precepts for the successful practice of homeopathy is the concern, the patience, the compassion and the empathy of the practitioner for the patient. This facet of homeopathy is often ignored, yet it ranks in importance next to the Laws of Similars, the minimum dose and treating the whole person. There is no place in homeopathy for the insensitive, brusque, domineering, impatient physician.

In a changing world, with its pollution, noise and increasing stress and with the emergence of new diseases, many of which are unconquered, there has never been a greater need for the homeopathic approach to medical treatment. I believe homeopathy will meet the challenge. Homeopathy must take a less defensive stance in the face of continuing opposition and adopt a more positive approach in declaring its undeniable benefits in the relief of suffering.

Trevor M. Cook

London/Las Vegas, 1988

CONTENTS

1 HISTORY AND DEVELOPMENT OF HOMEOPATHY

Homeopathy is as old as medicine itself. The basic precept of this system of medicine was recognized in ancient Greece by the physician Hippocrates (460-350 B.C.), who is generally regarded as the "Father of Medicine." He wrote: "By similar things a disease is produced and through the application of the like, it is cured." Hippocrates, in an oblique manner, recognized the natural ability of the body to cure itself in writing that medical treatment is aimed at "removing the impediments to people getting better." He also wrote of the symptoms of a disease as the expression of Nature's healing powers.

The Greek philosopher Aristotle (384-322 B.C.), who studied under Plato, also recognized the fundamental principle of homeopathy when, in one of his 22 surviving papers, he wrote, "Often the simile acts upon the simile." Like Hippocrates, however, he did not subject it to any scientific study to support the theory.

Second only to Hippocrates among the founders of medicine was another Greek physician, Galen (130-200 A.D.). Skilled in anatomy and physiology, he wrote of "natural cure by the likes." Galen was recognized as the authority in medicine for more than 1,000 years and, during this time, no significant progress was made.

During the 15th and 16th centuries, when medicine was developing slowly as a scientific study, the Swiss physician and leading medical reformer Theophrastus Bombastus von Hohenheim (1493-1541), who adopted the pseudonym Paracelsus, rejected the principle of opposite acting remedies and stated that "sames must be cured by sames." He also believed that every diseased organ had its corresponding remedy in Nature. Like his prede-

1

cessors, however, his reasoning was largely intuitive and lacked a precise scientific approach.

The first precise enunciation of the fundamental homeopathic principle was given in the early 17th century by a Danish physician, Dr. George Stahl, using the assumptions of Paracelsus. He wrote: "To treat with opposite acting remedies is the reverse of what it ought to be. I am convinced that disease will yield to, and be cured by, remedies that produce similar affections." Again, his views were not considered to have a scientific basis and were ignored by the medical profession, which relied largely on draconian, purgative methods of treatment, consisting of venesection or bloodletting, augmented by stomach-rending emetics, laxatives and massive doses of often poisonous medicines, many of which caused serious side effects.

William Harvey's (1578-1657) theory of the circulation of the blood was published in England in 1628. This fundamental discovery opened up the path to modern medicine as a whole.

FOUNDATION OF MODERN HOMEOPATHY

The basic concept of treating likes with likes, that is, using remedies which are capable of producing in a healthy person similar symptoms to those experienced in the patient, remained undeveloped. Although it had been known for some 2,000 years, it was never subjected to systematic, scientific study or used to any extent in practice: it remained simply the germ of an idea.

The founder of the modern system of homeopathic treatment was a brilliant German physician, Dr. Samuel Hahnemann.

Born April 10, 1755, in the town of Meissen in Saxony (now in East Germany), the second son of Christian Gottfried and Johanna Hahnemann, he was given the names Christian Friedrich Samuel. To avoid confusion with his father's name, he was called Samuel Hahnemann. His father was an artist of the famed Meissen porcelain.

A thin, delicate, fair-haired boy, Samuel Hahnemann was of a studious disposition. He led a disciplined boyhood where high moral standards, industry and piety prevailed under the guidance of his father. He was born into the Lutheran Protestant faith and retained a strong religious conviction all his life.

At the age of fifteen, Samuel moved from the Meissen Elementary School to the Prince's Grammar School,* where his exceptional academic ability was quickly recognized. He was a diligent student and, in later years, he wrote that he was "frequently ailing from overstudying." His schooling was often interrupted, however, as he was forced to work at menial tasks to help support his family. He displayed a gift for languages and, even at twelve years old, he taught younger boys Greek and Latin.

On graduating from the Prince's School in 1775, at the outbreak of the American War of Independence, Samuel Hahnemann entered the University of Leipzig to study medicine. He did not enjoy his student days, however, as he not only had to scrape a meager living by translating Greek and English into German for rich students, but, more importantly, because he quickly became disenchanted with his medical teaching methods and the lack of practice facilities.

Hahnemann took up the study of chemistry, which since his birth had taken a great leap forward as a distinct science. His contemporaries included Cavendish (1766, identification of gases in air); Priestley and Lavoisier (1770-1772, the nature of combustion); Priestley and Cavendish (1781-1785, composition of water); Proust, Dalton, Avogadro, Berzelius and others.

After only two years at Leipzig, a very frustrated Hahnemann, left the university and traveled to Vienna where he worked at a hospital to gain the practical experience he lacked. Subsequently, he went to Transylvania (now part of Romania), where he worked as a family physician and librarian to the Governor for a year. This gave him the opportunity to further his knowledge of botany and chemistry and to study more languages. By this time he was able to speak German, Latin, Greek, English, French and Spanish quite fluently.

In the spring of 1779, Hahnemann decided to complete his studies at the University of Erlangen in Bavaria. Erlangen un-

---

*The Burgermeister of Meissen wrote the author in 1981 that the Prince's School existed until 1941, and an Agricultural and Engineering College was founded on the site 12 years later. The house where Samuel Hahnemann was born has long since been demolished and the site is now crossed by a road extension. There is a commemorative plaque with a bust of Meissen's most famous son on the house nearest to the original site and a monument with a granite pedestal stands at the end of the Neumarkt, which was erected in 1958. There is another monument to Hahnemann in Leipzig. Some of Hahnemann's original letters, including his letter of thanks on being awarded the Freedom of the City of Meissen on his 86th birthday, are held in the Council archives.

doubtedly attracted him since it was one of the reformed, free-thinking universities of his time, were there was a critical reawakening socially, politically, spiritually and intellectually, in contrast to the old, narrow orthodox approach of the older universities. The awakening of this critical spirit matched Samuel Hahnemann's mood and character. He was awarded the degree of Doctor of Medicine on August 10, 1779 at the age of 24.

Medical Practice in the 18th Century

Samuel Hahnemann began his career as a practicing physician in Hettstedt, a small copper-mining town at the foot of the Hartz mountains. The squalid living conditions of the miners and their families, and his inability to provide effective and humane medical treatment to these poor people, fueled his frustration and despair.

Medical practice at that time was based on purging the disease from the body. Bloodletting, or venesection, was nothing short of a mania. The medical textbooks urged repeated, copious, venesections "until the patient faints," and even such conditions as whooping cough or pregnancy fell victim to the knife. Alternatively, dozens of blood-sucking leeches were applied to the affected parts. Other forms of purgation followed, including stomach-rending emetics, violent laxatives and enemas. Finally, if the patient had not succumbed from the treatment, massive doses of poisonous remedies were administered. Small wonder that Hahnemann believed that more people died of their treatment rather than their disease!

Nine months later, Hahnemann left for Dessau. He wrote at this time: "In Hettstedt it is impossible to develop either mentally or physically." Following the social custom in Germany in the late 18th century, Hahnemann was a regular visitor to the local pharmacy. It was here that he pursued his interest in chemistry and also met the stepdaughter of the apothecary owner, Johanna Kuchler, a pretty seventeen-year-old girl whom he was to marry a year later.

Hahnemann did not stay long in Dessau and soon moved to the small, rural town of Gommern. Although he enjoyed his family life with Johanna and their first-born daughter, Henriette, once again he was frustrated in his medical calling. The country folk of Gommern were superstitious and preferred to rely on their old quack remedies rather than a young doctor who was a stranger to them.

It was in Gommern that Hahnemann began to translate books to supplement his meager income. He also wrote his first medical essay, published in Leipzig in 1784, entitled, *Directions for Curing Old Diseases*. This essay clearly showed his growing disenchantment with medicine and the medical profession. This was his first criticism of medical practice, launching him on a crusade for medical reform, that was to continue for the rest of his life.

He stressed need for public hygiene, for fresh air, adequate sleep and regular exercise and a sensible diet. He proposed that houses be spaced apart, that they should be light and admit plenty of fresh air, and that sewage be properly treated. In all these things, he was years ahead of his time. It also presaged his life's mission to find a more humane and compassionate system of medicine and to fight for its acceptance in the face of ignorance, prejudice and reactionary forces. Another pattern of his future life began to evolve—that of constant wandering—when he moved to the ancient city of Dresden, the capital of Saxony.

In Dresden, Johanna gave birth to their first son, Friedrich, and Hahnemann renewed his studies in chemistry and medicine while translating books from French, English, Latin and Greek into his native German to augment his income. He soon made new friends, including Dr. Samuel Wagner, who when he became ill, recommended Hahnemann as his *locum tenens* (temporary replacement) as Medical Officer of Health for Dresden.

The wide-ranging responsibilities of this post gave the 33-year-old Hahnemann valuable experience. A few years later, he wrote a book, *The Friend of Health*, published in Leipzig in 1795, in which he drew on his experience in Dresden. After Dr. Wagner's death, he applied for the permanent post, but his application was unsuccessful.

Over four years in Dresden, Hahnemann translated five major books totaling 1,780 pages. In translating the books, he took the liberty of adding his own comments to the texts, which demonstrated *inter alia* his knowledge of chemistry and his distrust of pharmacists and the purity of the medicines they dispensed. He also wrote many articles on medicine and chemistry during this period and two books, one on arsenic poisoning and the other on the diagnosis and treatment of venereal disease. Both books were based on his work as Medical Officer and both books received good reviews.

At the end of 1789, having failed to gain the post he applied for, Hahnemann moved his family to Leipzig. By this time, he was disgusted with contemporary medical practice, which he saw as crude, barbaric and ineffectual. This view was to arouse the enmity of medical practitioners and bring suffering to him and his family.

The next five years saw the ever-growing Hahnemann family moving almost aimlessly from place to place. From Leipzig they moved to a village on the outskirts of the city, where the family, now seven, nearly starved, while Hahneman wrote by candlelight, behind a curtain in a corner of a single room, until the early hours of each morning. "I have entirely given up my practice for the past year," he wrote. "My daily bread is assured by my writing—I want a place where I can live quietly and privately and yet can enlarge my knowledge as a scholar . . . four daughters and one son together with my wife, constitute the spice of life."

First Proving—The Homeopathic Priniciple

It was during this difficult time that Hahnemann performed an epoch-making experiment that was to lay the foundation for his new system of medicine—homeopathy. It arose when he was translating from English into German a book written by a distinguished Scottish physician, William Cullen, *A Treatise on Materia Medica*. It was an account of a drug, cinchona or Peruvian Bark (Cortex Peruvianus), widely used for the treatment of malaria, first in South America and subsequently in Europe, which prompted the experiment.

For several days Hahnemann took large doses of the drug and carefully noted the symptoms he experienced. His feet and fingertips became cold, he became drowsy, his heart began to palpitate, his pulse quickened and he experienced trembling in all his limbs, a thirst and redness of cheeks. The symptoms lasted only for a few hours and recurred each time he repeated the dose. Thus, the drug Cinchona, *when taken by a healthy person*, induced symptoms similar to malaria—the very disease the drug was used to cure. Hahnemann noted in the book that "Cinchona bark, which is used as a remedy for intermittent fever [malaria], acts because it can produce symptoms similar to those of intermittent fever in healthy people." He had established the basic precept of homeopathy, foreshadowed by Hippocrates, Galen, Stahl and Paracelsus.

Apparently, he did not appreciate the full significance of his discovery at the time, because, in further annotations of Cullen's book, he reverted to his attacks on medical practice—bloodletting, fever remedies, weakening diet, everlasting aperients, clysters (enemas) and the like.

In spite of further public attacks on the medical profession, principally in the newspaper *Der Anzeiger*, published in Gotha, Hahnemann's contribution to science was recognized in 1791 by his election to the Leipzig Economical Society and the Academy of Science of Mainz. But the opposition to Hahnemann by the German physicians for his critical views was hardening.

In the spring of 1792, Hahnemann moved to the Principality of Gotha to take up a post as manager of an asylum for the insane. The offer probably arose through his friendship with the editor of *Der Anzeiger*, R.Z. Becker. Hahnemann's benefactor was Duke Ernst of Saxe-Coburg-Gotha, who provided his hunting lodge for the asylum. It was likely that the Duke's initiative was prompted by the insanity of an old acquaintance, Herr Klockenbring, a prominant politician in Hanover. In any event, Herr Klockenbring became Hahnemann's only patient.

True to his innovative approach, Hahnemann rejected the cruel treatment of the insane prevailing at that time. They were chained in dungeon-like cells, abused and whipped, only to be released on Sundays, when visitors to the "hospitals" and workhouses would prod and tease them to provoke reactions in their tortured minds as a form of amusement. Instead, Hahnemann developed a more compassionate treatment, building up a rapport with his patient and gaining his confidence. Again, he demonstrated that he was ahead of his time, and it is regretted that he did not have more opportunity with more patients to develop his methods.

His patient cured, Hahnemann moved north to Molschleben, where he resumed his literary work. His book, the *Pharmaceutical Lexicon*, in four volumes, broke new ground in the preparation of medicines. The procedures he described anticipated modern practices most accurately and many of his recommendations, including quality control, are now enshrined in Good Manufacturing Practice, generally recognized by most government bodies worldwide today.

The rejoicing at the birth of Hahnemann's second son, Ernst, was short-lived. The baby was killed when their coach overturned while journeying to their next home in Göttingen. Hahnemann and Johanna were to face further tragedies in the years to come when two of their daughters were murdered and their elder son became insane.

His wandering lifestyle continued for thirteen years, and he lived in twenty different towns with an ever-growing family. During this period, from 1793 until 1805, only Hahnemann's brilliant writings punctuated his progress. He wrote several essays, including *New Principles for Ascertaining the Curative Power of Drugs* and *Antidotes to Some Heroic Vegetable Substances.*

In his essay *New Principles for Ascertaining the Curative Power of Drugs,* published in *Hufeland's Medical Journal* in 1796, he wrote:

> One should proceed as rationally as possible by experiments of the medicines on the human body. Only by this means (provings) can the true nature, the real effect of the medicinal substance be discovered ... Every effective remedy incites in the human body an illness peculiar to itself ... One should imitate nature, which, at times, heals a chronic disease by an additional one. One should apply in the disease to be healed, particularly if chronic, that remedy which is liable to stimulate another artificially produced disease as similar as possible, and the former will be healed.

Simila Similibus—like with likes. That is, in order to cure disease, we must seek medicines that can excite similar symptoms in the healthy body.

Hahnemann's enunciation of the fundamental principle of homeopathy was thus written six years after his original experiments with Cinchona. Many homeopaths, therefore, date the birth of modern homeopathy as 1796. It was, however, only the beginning for Hahnemann and for homeopathy.

Immunology and Homeopathy

In that same year, 1796, Dr. Edward Jenner, a practicing physician in Gloucestershire, England, infected a young boy with cowpox by transferring the infection from a cowpox sore on the hand of a milkmaid to immunize him against the similar but deadly disease, smallpox, thus demonstrating the principle of immunization. Although it was a remarkable coincidence that Hahnemann introduced homeopathy in the same year, its close relationship with immunology is now clearly understood.

Like Hahnemann, Jenner's findings were opposed by sections of the medical profession. One even suggested that people vaccinated with cowpox serum would develop cow-like characteristics! Drawing on his own experience, Hahnemann was quick to recognize Dr. Jenner's predicament. He wrote to his friend Dr. Stapf: "Dr. Jenner's vaccination against smallpox has proved itself everywhere, yet, in England, so many attacks in print were issued against it that at one time I counted twenty. . . ."

Hahnemann continued his journeys and and his writing. Between 1797 and 1810, he wrote the following: *Some Kinds of Remittent Fevers* (1797); *Cure and Prevention of Scarlet Fever* (1801); *A New Alkali Salt, Alkali Pneum* (1801); *On the Power of Small Doses of Medicine in General and Belladonna In Particular* (1801); *Coffee and Its Effects* (1803); *Aesculapius in the Balance* (1805); and *Observations on the Brown's Elements of Medicine* (1810). These essays were particularly significant since they included many separate statements which collectively made up the elements of homeopathy. Clearly, his new concept of medicine, including his belief in small doses, were formulating in Hahnemann's mind as a coherent system. Only his essay on the new alkaline salt proved erroneous, and Hahnemann readily admitted his mistake. This mistake was promptly seized upon by certain members of the medical profession to discredit his accurate and brilliant observations in his other essays.

The Organon of the Healing Art

Torgau, on the River Elbe, was the location for Hahnemann's next "sojourn," as he called it. He arrived there early in 1805 and continued his writings. Several published essays culminated in the publication of his quintessential work, the *Organon of Rational Medicine (Organon der Rationellen Heilkunde)*, by Arnold of Dresden in 1810. Later he revised the title of the book, to the *Organon of the Healing Art*.

Today, the *Organon* is still universally recognized as the authoritative statement on the practice of homeopathy. It has been published in six editions and translated into ten languages. The basic principle of homeopathy, which Hahnemann expanded into *Similia Similibus Curentur* (Let likes be treated with likes), and this "Law of Similars," as it is known, is immutable. Hahnemann wrote his own definition of cure in the *Organon*:

"The physician's high and only mission is to restore the sick to health, to cure as it is termed.

"The highest ideal of cure is the speedy, gentle and enduring restoration of health, of the removal and annihilation of disease in its entirety by the quickest most trustworthy and least harmful way according to principles that can be readily understood.

"Every medicine, which among the symptoms it can cause in a healthy body, reproduces those most present in a given disease, is capable of curing the disease in the swiftest, most thorough and most enduring fashion."

In the winter of 1810-1811, while the criticism of Hahnemann's *Organon* was growing among the medical establishment, Napoleon Bonaparte was preparing his conquest of Russia. His strategy involved the building of a defensive line along the course of the River Elbe to keep a route open from Danzig, where his troops were held, to Russia. Torgau was heavily fortified and huge ramparts were constructed to protect the bridge* across the river.

These warlike activities unsettled Hahnemann and, after an unsuccessful attempt to gain a post at the University of Göttingen, he moved once again, this time back to Leipzig. He was beginning the most turbulent and acrimonious periods in his life. Personal tragedy, war and persecution for his beliefs surrounded him for the next fifteen years.

Anxious to build up a following for his new medical doctrine, he attempted to set up a college for the postgraduate study of homeopathy, but failed to attract a single physician. His next move was to gain a professional post at the University of Leipzig. In this he was successful after delivering a masterly dissertation on the White Hellebore (Veratrum Album), avoiding any contentious allusion to homeopathy.

From the winter of 1812, Hahnemann gave two lectures a week in which he regularly berated conventional medical practice. Since these unconstructive, almost uncontrollable, outbursts usually followed mention of the value of homeopathy, it won him few supporters and many professional enemies.

His university lectures were interrupted when, in October 1813, the Battle of Leipzig, between the armies of Napoleon and the Allied nations, was fought over three days in and around the

---

*It was at the center of this same bridge in Torgau, 134 years later—on April 25, 1945—that American and Russian soldiers linked hands to mark the end of World War II in Europe.

city. The holocaust left 80,000 soldiers dead and similar number wounded. Every available physician in Leipzig, including Hahnemann, worked day and night treating the wounded in makeshift military hospitals.

An outbreak of typhus in the city following the battle gave Hahnemann his first opportunity to give a clear demonstration of the efficacy of homeopathic treatment. The results were published in a German newspaper a year later and they showed that out of a total of 180 patients treated homeopathically, only two died. The mortality rate by conventional treatment at that time was more than 50 percent!

During the next few years, Hahnemann's medical practice flourished, and the success of his homeopathic treatment encouraged a small, dedicated band of young physicians to gather around him. He enjoyed a happy family life, with regular meetings in his house of groups of physicians who responded to his wit and wisdom and avidly sought to learn more about homeopathy. From this group he formed a network of collaborators to carry out provings of new homeopathic medicines at great risk to themselves.

Materia Medica Pura

The results of these provings were published in Hahnemann's *Materia Medica Pura*. Between 1811 and 1821, six volumes of this important book were published. Apart from a detailed account of each homeopathic medicine and its application in the treatment of disease, he elaborated on the personalized approach to homeopathic prescribing. He instructed:

"It is the duty of physicians to distinguish subtle variations of every *individual* case—that is to specialize and individualize in each personal case, instead of treating the disease.

"There is no case of dynamic disease which will not be rapidly and permanently cured in no more easy, rapid, certain, reliable and permanent manner by any conceivable method of treatment other than by means of homeopathic medicine in small doses," he maintained.

The *Materia Medica Pura* even today is standard reference work for homeopaths worldwide, and together with his *Organon of Rational Healing*, constitutes the basis of any study of homeopathy.

Shortly after the death of Hahnemann's daughter Wilhelmina, the campaign by the medical establishment against homeopathy began in earnest. A number of highly critical articles on the subject were followed by a formal complaint by the apothecaries of Leipzig, accusing Hahnemann of infringing on their rights by preparing his own homeopathic medicines. Hahnemann presented his own defense in the court. He reasoned that homeopathic medicines were only simple medicines and not compounds of several ingredients and the word "dispensing" did not apply. Furthermore, he argued that the very small doses employed in homeopathy, so small that the active ingredients could not be detected, would warrant no fee from the apothecary, since the law said that they should charge by weight. His defense failed, however, and the court of Leipzig imposed a fine on Hahnemann. The court also forbade him to prepare his own medicines.

Another episode concerning Hahnemann's treatment of Prince Karl of Schwarzenburg, the commander of the Allied forces at the Battle of Leipzig, fueled the mounting resentment of the Leipzig physicians. The Prince, a powerful and famous figure throughout Europe, had suffered a stroke and, when conventional treatment failed, traveled with his entourage from his native Austria to Leipzig to receive treatment at the hands of the now famous Dr. Hahnemann.

Unfortunately, the Prince's drinking habit coupled with copious venesections carried out by his allopathic physicians, led to his death. Fortunately Hahnemann had already given up the case.

The allopathic physicians, jealous of Hahnemann being chosen by Prince Karl, now seized upon his death to discredit homeopathy. The Prince's postmortem report included a vicious attack on homeopathy and claimed that it was positively harmful because it delayed "strong measures."

This was only the first of many acrimonious and bitter attacks on Hahnemann. He was ostracized by many of his students who feared that their association with him and homeopathy would spoil their chances of gaining their medical degrees. Articles ridiculing homeopathy appeared regularly in the newspapers and medical journals. In this atmosphere, and having been denied the preparation of the medicines, Hahnemann found it almost impossible to practice.

Mark Twain, a keen homeopath, could have had Hahnemann in mind when he wrote: "The man with new idea is a crank, until his idea succeeds."

Other homeopathic physicians were also persecuted. Dr. Karl Franz was forced to retire and Dr. Christian Hornburg's homeopathic medicines were confiscated and buried symbolically in a local churchyard. Dr. Hornburg became the first martyr for homeopathy when, after being hauled before the courts on several occasions, he was eventually imprisoned and died three days later.

The final blow came when thirteen Leipzig physicians published a long article in the *Leipziger Zeitung* refuting claims made by Hahnemann in an earlier article (In fact, they totally misunderstood Hahnemann's excellent article). Meanwhile, the Leipzig apothecaries began further attempts to force Hahnemann to give up his practice. In spite of belated support for him in a protest against his treatment signed by forty local residents, Hahnemann left Leipzig in June, 1821 for Köthen.

He did not want to live in the small town of Köthen, but the ruler of the Principality, Duke Ferdinand, gave him permission to practice homeopathy freely. Indeed, the Duke was Hahnemann's first patient there! Hahnemann was now 66 years old and wished for nothing more than to continue to practice his new therapy quietly without further hindrance.

Indeed, his wishes were fulfilled and, with the assistance of his daughters, Charlotte and Louise, his practice flourished. Not only this, but news of his spectacular successes with homeopathic treatment won many adherents, both lay and professional throughout Europe. He corresponded regularly with his many professional disciples practicing homeopathy elsewhere, in particular with his close friend Johann Stapf, Carl Bonninghausen and Constantine Hering. Many of his letters were animated discussions of different aspects of homeopathy.

In 1812, Hahnemann's last major book was published, *Chronic Diseases: Their Peculiar Nature and Their Homeopathic Cure.* The first volume expanded on the principles and practice of homeopathy and its wholistic approach, that is, the treatment of the whole person. The second volume referred to the "vital force" to describe the inherited natural curative power of the human body. He wrote: "It is certain that the vital forces may achieve victory over disease, without inflicting losses on the body, provided they are assisted and directed in their action by a properly selected homeopathic remedy."

In emphasizing the vital force, Hahnemann introduced the metaphysical aspects of homeopathy, which was a departure from the essentially scientific approach in his earlier works. Further, he introduced the "psora theory," a latent predisposition to disease handed down from generation to generation. Unfortunately, his attempts to describe the meaning of homeopathy caused considerable division and criticism from the homeopaths themselves. Hahnemann's more contentious theories, however, are thought to be a manifestation of his deeply held conviction that God had provided the means for mankind to be relieved from suffering.

HOMEOPATHIC TREATMENT OF CHOLERA

During the winter of 1831–1832, a cholera epidemic swept through Europe from Russia to the Atlantic shores. Conventional medical treatment proved to be virtually ineffective and the disease claimed several hundred thousand lives. In the latter part of 1831, Hahnemann wrote four essays, on the nature of cholera and its homeopathic treatment, which he had published in four different cities to ensure they would not all be suppressed. He described a preventive and a curative treatment based on a careful analysis of the symptoms of the disease. He advised Camphor, given prophylactically, followed by Cuprum Metallicum and Rhus Toxicodendron, then Bryonia alba and Veratrum album given alternately.

Hahnemann's homeopathic treatment proved remarkably successful. For example, in the Hungarian town of Raab, only six patients of 154 treated homeopathically died (less than 4 percent), whereas 50 percent of 821 patients treated conventionally died. Similar results were obtained in several cities throughout Europe where homeopathy was practiced.

At this time the medical profession was totally ignorant of the existence of the disease virus and the value of cleanliness and disinfection in checking the spread of disease. Yet, in one of his essays, Hahnemann wrote: "In order to render the spread of cholera impossible, the garments, linen, etc. of all strangers must be quarantined (whilst their bodies are cleansed with baths) and heated for two hours at a stove heat of 80°C.—this represents the temperature at which all known infections and consequently the living miasms, are annihilated. . . .*cholera infection is most probably caused by a swarm of infinitely small, invisible living organisms* so murderously hostile to human life."

Once again Hahnemann was years ahead of his contemporaries.

New Lease on Life

By 1835, Hahnemann had virtually retired from practice. His beloved wife for nearly fifty years, Johanna, had died five years earlier and he now spent his days writing, sitting in his garden and receiving an occasional visitor. This period, however, proved to be only the prelude to the final chapter in his life. His new life began with a visit to Köthen by a young Parisienne named Melanie D'Hervilly. Ostensibly she had come to receive homeopathic treatment from the celebrated Dr. Samuel Hahnemann but, after she had stayed in the town for a few months, their engagement was announced. They were married quietly in the front room of Hahnemann's home in January, 1835.

To the anguish of Hahnemann's unmarried daughters Charlotte and Louise, who still lived with their father, the newly married couple—she at the age of about 30 and he at 80—left for a new life in Paris. Only three months before, on his 80th birthday, Hahnemann had been elected an Honorary Member of the North American Academy of Homeopathic Healing Art in Allentown, Pennsylvania, the first college of Homeopathy to be established in the United States.

Within two years of moving to Paris, Hahnemann, driven by Melanie's personality and social ambitions, set up a practice in a spacious mansion on the Rue de Milan. His remarkable success with his homeopathic treatment, coupled with public-relations style promotion of his work by Melanie soon made his practice the most celebrated throughout France, then Europe, and the rest of the world. People from all walks of life flocked to his door, rich and poor alike, and none was turned away.

The First Homeopathic Hospital

Hahnemann wrote to his friend Dr. Bonninghausen in 1831: "If only we had a homeopathic hospital, with a teacher who could instruct students in the practice of homeopathy." His wish was fulfilled two years later when the first homeopathic hospital was opened in Leipzig. The hospital was established in a house purchased with the funds collected at Hahnemann's Doctorate Jubilee, held in 1829, and incorporated a dispensary, a library and twenty beds. Its first director, Dr. Moritz Müller, was an able physician and administrator.

In spite of an auspicious beginning, the hospital was finally closed, after much confusion and acrimony, ten years later. Regretably, it was Hahnemann himself whose autocratic behavior was the prime factor in its closure. Incensed by an article by Dr. Müller in which he put forward the view that homeopathy and allopathy were not mutually exclusive, Hahnemann publicly declared his displeasure even before the opening ceremony. The article, entitled *A Word to the Half-Homeopaths of Leipzig,* appeared in the *Leipziger Tageblatt* and was a bitter condemnation of those physicians who practiced both homeopathy and allopathy. Not surprisingly, Dr. Müller resigned as director. His successor resigned when Hahnemann, on his only visit to the hospital, disbanded the Board of Directors and assumed responsibility for its management. Acrimony, financial difficulty and the inability of Hahnemann, aged 80 and living two days' coach–ride away in Köthen, to exercise proper control, finally caused the hospital to close its doors in October 1842.

By the early 1840s the bastions of allopathic opposition had fallen and homeopathy was inexorably moving forward, establishing itself in country after country and growing in its popularity.

DEATH OF SAMUEL HAHNEMANN

After a short illness, Samuel Hahnemann's long life came peacefully to its close in the early hours of July 2, 1843, in his 90th year. Attended only by his wife, Melanie, his daughter, Amalie, and his grandson, Leopold Suss-Hahnemann,* he was buried in a public grave in Montmartre Cemetery in Paris.

*A year after the publication of my biography of Samuel Hahnemann, in 1981, I was approached by William Herbert Tankard of Crowborough in England. Mr. Tankard had known for some time that he was descended from Samuel Hahnemann. He remembered his grandmother, Amalie, telling him, as a young boy, of her visits to "Uncle Leo" at Ventnor on the Isle of Wight, and it was on reading the book that his interest in his illustrious forbear was aroused.

"Uncle Leo" was Hahnemann's grandson, the only son of his daughter Amalie (1789-1881). Leopold Suss-Hahnemann emigrated to England after qualifying in medicine at the University of Leipzig, and practiced homeopathy in London until his retirement, when he settled in the Isle of Wight. He died there in 1914, shortly before the outbreak of World War I.

Leopold's youngest daughter by his first wife, Amalia Spavin, was William Tankard's grandmother, Amalia Elise Sugden, and she had two children, Winifred Maud (born in 1898), and Herbert Cyril (born in 1900). Winifred married William Percy Tankard, and their son, William Herbert, was born in January, 1902.

William Herbert Tankard is the great-great-great-grandson of Samuel Hahnemann. He served as a Captain in the British Army in World War II, a Lloyd's underwriter and he is a Freeman of the City of London. Now in his late 60s, Mr. Tankard and his wife Elizabeth have several grandchildren. In 1982, Mr. and Mrs. Tankard were elected honorary life members of The Hahnemann Society, and in 1988 he was elected a Life Fellow of the U.K.H.M.A.

Why Melanie consigned her husband's body to a near-pauper's grave without pomp and ceremony has never been revealed. Possibly, it was her way of snubbing all those who had persecuted him throughout his professional life.

His disciples and admirers were not to be thwarted, however. On March 24, 1898, Hahnemann's body was exhumed in the presence of leaders of the Central Homeopathic Commission, the French Homeopathic Society, the Society of Homeopathic Physicians of Rhineland and Westphalia, the British Homeopathic Society (later the Faculty of Homeopathy), the American Institute of Homeopathy and other representatives from nearly 50 countries. Hahnemann's grandson, Dr. Leopold Suss-Hahnemann, and other members of the Hahnemann family were also present. After long speeches by civic dignitaries, the coffin was borne through the center of Paris, followed by a long procession of coaches, to the Père Lachaise Cemetery, where the most renowned people of France are buried. His remains had at last found a final resting place.

Two years later, through the generosity of American homeopathic physicians, a 14-foot-high granite monument was erected over the grave. Some time later another inscription was added to the monument in accordance with Hahnemann's last wish. *Non inutilis vixi*—"I have not lived in vain."

Samuel Hahnemann had endured personal tragedy and had fought against the implacable persecution of a bigoted, prejudiced and reactionary medical establishment for most of his life. He lived to see his fight for medical reform and his gentle, compassionate approach to medicine firmly established. At the same time, his dogmatic and inflexible attitude in his later years left a legacy of conflict for future generations.

A year after Hahnemann's death, in 1844, an American dentist, Horace Wells, had a tooth extracted under nitrous oxide for the first time. The gas had been discovered in 1776 by Thomas Beddoes, while Hahnemann was studying at Leipzig. This was the beginning of modern anesthetics. A year later another American dentist in Boston anesthetized a patient with ether for the

---

"Toby" Tankard's most treasured possessions are a gold signet ring bearing Hahnemann's seal, and a silver coin presented to Hahnemann at the Jubilee Celebration of his doctorate, in Köthen on August 10, 1829.

The inscription reads: "Samuel Hahnemann Natus Misanen D.X. Aprilis MDCCLV Doct. Creat. Erlangus. D.X. Augusti MDCCLXXI."

removal of a tumor. Chloroform also came into use, followed by ethyl chloride, cyclopropane, cocaine and novocaine (1903).

Louis Pasteur announced his discovery of the cause of fermentation in alcohol and milk at the École Normale in France in 1857. Pasteur's identification of atmospheric organisms stimulated the work of Joseph Lister (1827-1912). He was the first to introduce antiseptics in the treatment of wounds.

None of these advances in conventional medical treatment was inconsistent with homeopathic concepts, but the antipathy toward homeopathy on the part of allopaths continue unabated. During a cholera outbreak in Great Britain in 1854, only 16.4 percent of the patients in the Royal London Homeopathic Hospital died, compared with an average mortality rate of 51.8 percent in other hospitals. Yet the report on this success was deliberately suppressed. The success of homeopathic treatment of cholera in an earlier epidemic, which swept Europe in 1831, was also ignored by the allopaths.

Nevertheless, homeopathy continued to prosper. At the turn of the century it had reached its zenith; it was being practiced in more than 60 countries worldwide, including France, Great Britain, United States, Canada, Italy, Sweden, Denmark, Austria, Norway, Holland, Ghana, South Africa, Kenya, Brazil, Argentina, Venezuela, Mexico, India, Sri Lanka, Australia, New Zealand and Russia.

It is estimated that about 400 million people were receiving homeopathic treatment during that time. In all these countries, homeopathic hospitals and medical schools were being established and medical associations were being formed. Indeed, in many countries, homeopathy had become the form of medicine preferred by the majority. Many homeopathic medicines were now included in the official Pharmacopoeias of many countries, yet homeopathy was still opposed by the medical establishment.

Throughout its history, homeopathy has been supported by many renowned people, including:

Royalty H.M. Queen Elizabeth II, H.M. King George VI, H.M. King George V, H.R.H. Prince Charles of Great Britain, Constantine XIII of Greece, King Haakon VII of Norway, King Peter II of Yugoslavia, Prince Karl of Austria.

Politicians Benjamin Disraeli; Mahatma Gandhi; Abraham Lincoln.

Musicians Sir Yehudi Menuhin, Sir Adrian Boult

Poets Johann Wolfgang von Goethe, Robert Browning.

Artists Sir Edwin Landseer, Édouard Manet
Writers Mark Twain, William Makepeace Thackeray,
Charles Dickens.
Actors Steve McQueen, Stewart Granger, Susan Hampshire,
Jack Warner
Scientists Marie Curie
Generals Duke of Wellington, Korsakov
Philanthropist John D. Rockefeller

The Decline of Homeopathy

The so-called miracle drug revolution began in 1909, with the discovery by Paul Ehrlich of the first specific anti-bacterial drug, Salvarsan, a synthetic, organo-arsenic compound for the treatment of syphilis. The race was on. In Paris, the activity of sulfanilamide, a product of the rising German dye industry, was shown to be active. A year later, in 1936, the British discoveries of the therapeutic activity of sulfathiazole, led the way to the discovery of a whole range of sulfonamide drugs. The introduction of amphetamines and barbiturate drugs soon followed. The first antibiotic, penicillin, was discovered by Alexander Fleming in 1928, and its therapeutic use was developed by H.W. Florey and E.B. Chain at Oxford in 1938.

In the euphoria at this time, it was thought that it was only a matter of time before every disease suffered by mankind for centuries past would be conquered. Dazzled by the apparent success of these wonder drugs, the physicians turned from homeopathy and its decline was accelerated.

Unfortunately, another factor contributed to the decline of homeopathy. A serious rift had developed in the profession between those physicians who followed the teachings of Dr. Richard Hughes in England and adherents of Dr. James Kent and H.C. Allen in America. The English school rejected the psora theory and other metaphysical ideas of Hahnemann in his later years, and laid emphasis on the modern scientific basis of homeopathy. Hughes believed that pathological symptoms and their modalities were more important than the mental symptoms and he only prescribed low potencies. Potencies higher than 30CH, above the Avagadro Limit, were dismissed by him as "airy nothings."

The American school rejected the dominance of medicine by technology. Preeminence was given to constitutional prescribing, believing that certain types of people have a special affinity for a particular drug and will respond positively to it for most conditions. The Kentists also prescribed very high potencies of 1M (1,000), 10M (10,000), and CM (100,000). They regarded the low potencies prescribed by the Hughesian homeopaths as close to allopathic dosages. Drs. Margaret Tyler, John Weir and Margery Blackie became devoted followers of the Kentist approach in England.

This schism within homeopathy provided the medical establishment of the day with more ammunition to discredit homeopathy. Another factor which contributed to the decline of homeopathy was the lack of research, which prevented it from keeping pace with scientific and medical developments. The multi-national pharmaceutical companies were pouring billions of dollars into research and development, whereas homeopathy had no such support.

Revival of Homeopathy

The renewed interest in homeopathy worldwide began in the late 1960s and, over the last twenty years, it has regained its rightful place as an intrinsic part of the whole fabric of modern medicine. There are many contributing factors in the great revival of homeopathy:

1. The increasing concern over the serious side effects of many modern drugs, which has led to their removal from the market, or their supply being severely restricted. In many cases, long-term side effects did not become apparent until these drugs had been prescribed and used for many years.

2. The addictive nature of many prescribed drugs.

3. Certain disease organisms have become impervious to drug treatment. For example, at one time it was thought that the antibiotic treatment of sexually transmitted diseases, such as gonorrhea, could guarantee a cure in one dose. Unfortunately the gonococcus has proved to be a versatile organism and, in the face of the uncontrolled use of antibiotics such as penicillin and tetracycline, it steadily became resistant to treatment. In spite of increasing the dose of penicillin, or adding a drug which slowed the removal of the antibiotic from the body, in certain parts of the world, single-dose penicillin treatment could no longer be guaranteed. If all the gonococci are not killed by antibiotic treatment, those that remain are stimulated to undergo mutations, resulting in increased resistance.

4. The rise in the incidence of old and new diseases, many

resulting from the hazards of living in the modern society. AIDS and many forms of cancer and heart disease have yet to be conquered.

5. Increasing health consciousness by the general public exemplified by the popularity of health foods, concern about all forms of pollution and a desire for the natural rather than the synthetic.

6. A growing number of people who reject the use of animals in medical research.

7. The increased desire of people to be treated as people and not as disease bearers.

8. The high cost of modern drugs.

It is not surprising, therefore, that more and more people are seeking alternative therapy. Homeopathic medicine meets all the requirements. With a track record proven over 180 years, homeopathy is a natural medicine which is safe, and has no side effects. Nonaddictive, it does not require animal experiments (only proving on healthy people). It is relatively inexpensive and it treats the whole person.

HOMEOPATHY IN THE UNITED STATES

Homeopathy arrived in the United States when Dr. Hans Burch Gram, the son of a Danish sea captain, set up practice in New York in 1828—at least 10 years before homeopathy crossed the few miles of the English Channel to Great Britain.

It was Dr. Constantine Hering who was the true architect of the development of homeopathy across the nation. Like Samuel Hahnemann, a native of Saxony, Constantine Hering was born in the town of Oschatz, on January 1, 1800. He studied medicine at the University of Leipzig.

In his final year, he was instructed by his tutor to write a thesis refuting the principles of homeopathy, but his study of the subject only convinced him of its worth. He wrote to Hahnemann to explain his predicament. The master replied that he should keep his belief in homeopathy to himself until he gained his degree and then practice homeopathy as he wished. Hering's commitment to homeopathy was so strong, however, that he refused to complete his thesis and moved to the University of Würzburg where, in 1826, he gained his Doctorate of Medicine.

For five years Hering traveled throughout South America, where he proved several new homeopathic medicines, including Lachesis, Spigelia and Theridion. He corresponded regularly with Samuel Hahnemann on homeopathic matters and they became close friends.

Dr. Hering emigrated to the United States in 1833, and within a year he had gathered a number of German immigrant physicians around him to establish a homeopathic infrastructure. First, he set up the North American Academy of Homeopathic Healing Art in Allentown, Pennsylvania, assisted by Drs. Detweiler, Bute, Ihm and Freitag, all German immigrants. His next step was the founding of the American Institute of Homeopathy, and he was elected its first President. The A.I.H. is the oldest medical professional body in the United States today. In 1836, Hering established a second teaching institution, the Homeopathic Medical College of Pennsylvania, which merged with the Hahnemann Medical College in 1880, by which time homeopathy was sweeping across America.

Another giant of American homeopathy was Dr. Detweiler who, in 1828, became the first physician to use homeopathy in Pennsylvania, where he practiced for the rest of his life.

Dr. James Tyler Kent, whose *Repertory* became a standard reference work, was born on March 31, 1849. He was a graduate of the Hahnemann College in Philadelphia, and subsequently taught at the Homeopathic College of St. Louis and Chicago. His teachings on the use of high potencies caused a rift with homeopathic physicians who favored low potencies (see Chapter 2). Dr. Kent died in Chicago in 1916.

A yellow fever epidemic in the southern states in the 1860s provided the opportunity to demonstrate the curative powers of homeopathic treatment. New homeopathic medical schools and hospitals were springing up from New York to San Francisco, until by 1900 there were 22 medical schools and nearly 100 hospitals where homeopathy was practiced exclusively. The first medical school for women was established in 1838. Approximately 6,000 physicians (about 25 percent), now practiced homeopathy. Homeopathic pharmacies existed in every major city. The first of these was established in Philadelphia in 1835 by William Boericke. Other pharmacies, which still flourish today, include Hermann Lutyies (1853) and Humphrey's (1854). The first pharmacy in California was established by Boericke and Runyon in 1870, but sadly it finally closed in 1981.

From the peak of its popularity in the early 1900s, homeopathy, as in Europe, declined rapidly in the United States. Five medical colleges closed in the early 1920s, the Hahnemann Medical College closed in 1940, and the last homeopathic hospital was closed in 1953. By 1960, only 100 physicians practiced homeopathy.

The massive revival of homeopathy which began in the early 1970s has not faltered. More and more physicians are turning to homeopathy, together with several thousand chiropractors, acupuncturists and naturopaths, who have combined their own disciplines with homeopathy to broaden their holistic approach. The mainstay of homeopathy in the United States, The National Center for Homeopathy, continues to provide courses for both professional and lay people, and many new homeopathic associations have been formed, including the Arizona Homeopathic Medical Association (1981), the Florida Homeopathic Association and the Homeopathic Association of Greater Chicago (1985).

The Society for Ultramolecular Medicine was formed in 1983, to bridge the gap between homeopathy and acupuncture. This society, which also embraces electrodiagnosis, is the sister organization to the Société Médicale de Biothérapie in Paris.

The acceptance of homeopathy varies from state to state in the United States. In Arizona, for example, the State Legislature gave its approval for the full recognition of homeopathy in 1986 for ten years, yet in the same year, the North Carolina Board of Medical Examiners revoked the license of a fully qualified physician, Dr. George Guess, for practicing homeopathy. Only three States—Arizona, Connecticut and Nevada—wholly recognize homeopathy.

The Food and Drug Administration has ruled that the important remedy Gelsemium sempervirens can only be supplied on prescription. In Pennsylvania, Apis mellifica was impounded as it did not show the indication for use on the label, and in Louisiana homeopathic remedies were banned because they were labeled in Latin!

The National Center for Homeopathy in Washington D.C., is leading the fight for the universal recognition of homeopathy, supported by the growing number of people who are receiving homeopathic treatment. The 42nd Congress of the International Homeopathic Medical League L.M.H.I. was held in Washington, D.C., in 1987, and was attended by over 300 physicians from 20 countries.

The American spelling of the healing art is *Homeopathy*.

Until 1986, the National Center for Homeopathy used the original spelling *Homoeopathy*, when the diphthong was removed because it was considered to be archaic. In spite of the difficulties, there is no reason to suppose that homeopathy will not continue to flourish in the United States on a scale not seen since the last century.

HOMEOPATHY IN GREAT BRITAIN

Homeopathy as introduced in Great Britain by Dr. Frederick Hervey Foster Quin, when he set up practice in King Street in London in 1832. The illegitimate son of the Duchess of Devonshire, he attended school in Putney and studied medicine at the University of Edinburgh. He gained his Doctorate of Medicine in 1819 at the age of 20.

Dr. Quin was appointed physician to Napoleon in exile, but Napoleon died before he took up the post. So instead, Dr. Quin left England for Europe, where he met Samuel Hahnemann in Köthen in 1826, and again several years later. On his second visit, he stayed to study homeopathy under the tutelage of the master. After serving as physician to the future King Leopold of Belgium and his family, he returned to England and set up a homeopathic practice.

Quin was a great wit and raconteur, as well as an accomplished physician, and his practice flourished, attracting such notables as Dickens, Thackeray and Disraeli. He also write several books and papers on the homeopathic treatment of cholera.

In 1844, Dr. Quin established, and became the first president of, the British Homeopathic Society, which in 1943 was renamed the Faculty of Homeopathy. The Faculty, with its offices in Great Ormond Street, London, had powers conferred on it under the Faculty of Homeopathy Act, 1950. Postgraduate courses in homeopathic medicine, open to registered medical practitioners, are run by the Faculty between October and May each year. The British Medical Council still does not recognize the Faculty Diploma.

Following the rapid growth of homeopathy throughout Britain between 1850 and 1900, several homeopathic hospitals were opened. The first—The London Homeopathic Hospital (later the Royal London Homeopathic Hospital)—was founded in Golden Square by Dr. Quin on Hahnemann's birthday in 1850. In 1859, the hospital moved to its present site in Great Ormond Street.

The original Liverpool Homeopathic Dispensaries were merged to form the Liverpool Hahnemann Hospital in 1887. The hospital was closed in 1976.

A dispensary set up by a number of homeopathic physicians in 1880 led to the establishment of the Glasgow Homeopathic Hospital, now situated in Great Western Road. A major research center, the Glasgow hospital also runs postgraduate courses for qualified practitioners of homeopathy. The Bristol Homeopathic Hospital was founded in 1883. Now situated on a hill in Cotham overlooking the city, the hospital still functions as a major center for homeopathic treatment in Britain. The Tunbridge Wells Homeopathic Hospital was originally a dispensary established in 1863. The present hospital was opened in Church Road in 1890. Homeopathic treatment is available as part of the National Health Service at all these hospitals. In recent years attempts to close or restrict their facilities have been strenuously resisted.

In the latter part of the 19th century, homeopathy in Britain was dominated by the powerful character and intellect of Dr. Richard Hughes. While accepting Hahnemann's concept of matching the totality of symptoms, he recognized that pathological symptoms and their modalities were important. Hughes also prescribed only low potencies, usually 6x, 12x and 6CH, but never higher than 30CH, in contrast with the high potencies favored by the American school led by Dr. James Tyler Kent. (See Chapter 4.)

At the height of the support for homeopathy in 1902, the British Homeopathic Association was founded. Although membership includes physicians, it was formed primarily to give the lay public in Britain a voice. The B.H.A. holds regular meetings, seminars and first-aid courses. The Hahnemann Society, which also seeks to educate the public and promote the study and practice of homeopathy, was formed by Dr. Alva Benjamin in 1958. It now has nearly 4,000 members.

Homeopathy has benefited from the support of the royal family in Britain over six generations. The author's researches in 1980 revealed that the first royal patron of homeopathy was Queen Adelaide, wife of King William IV. A German princess whose family had been treated homeopathically all her life, she summoned Dr. Johann Stapf, a disciple of Samuel Hahnemann, to Windsor Castle in 1835, thereby establishing a family tradition.

Queen Adelaide (who gave her name to the Australian city) was the aunt of Prince Albert of Saxe-Coburg-Gotha, whose father was Hahnemann's benefactor at the Asylum. Prince Albert married Queen Victoria in 1840.

King George VI (1895-1952) was a dedicated believer in the benefits of homeopathy. He appointed Dr. John Weir (1879-1971, later Sir John) as his homeopathic physician after his coronation in 1937. He was so impressed with his treatment that he named one of his racehorses Hypericum. It went on to win the English Classic race, the 2,000 Guineas, at Newmarket in 1946. On the day of the King's funeral in 1952, five kings and three queens received homeopathic treatment for bereavement.

In 1969, Sir John Weir was succeeded by Dr. Margery Blackie, the first woman to hold the position as homeopathic physician to the British monarch. Today, H.M. Queen Elizabeth II, H.M. Queen Elizabeth the Queen Mother, H.R.H. Prince Charles and other members of the Royal Family give their patronage to homeopathic medicine.

Since the mid-1970s the number of people receiving homeopathic treatment in Britain has trebled. A survey conducted by the Institute for Complementary Medicine (the modern approach is to regard homeopathy as complementary to conventional medicine, rather than as an alternative medicine) showed that the number of homeopathic patients exceeds one million and is increasing by 15 to 20 percent each year.

This growth is manifested in the spontaneous formation of over 60 local and regional lay homeopathic groups or societies throughout Britain since 1974. The largest of these organizations is the North West Friends of Homeopathy under the chairmanship of Mrs. Hilda Jackson. In 1983, most of these organizations banded together to form the National Association of Homeopathic Groups, with the aim of coordinating their efforts.

The growth of homeopathy is also demonstrated by the fact that, in 1977, only five pharmacies stocked homeopathic medicines; today, there are 5,000. Homeopathic medicines are available by prescription under the National Health Service.

Other organizations formed in recent years include the British Association of Homeopathic Pharmacists (1980), the British Association of Homeopathic Veterinary Surgeons (1981)—now with more than 100 members—and the United Kingdom Homeopathic Medical Association (1986). The Hahnemann College of Homeopathy, which comes under the aegis of the latter Association, provides courses for physicians, osteopaths, acupuncturists and paramedics and has recently set up postgraduate studies.

HOMEOPATHY IN FRANCE

In no country has homeopathy flourished more than in France where, according to a recent survey, more than a quarter of the population are treated regularly or occasionally with homeopathic remedies.

Even before Dr. Samuel Hahnemann set up his practice in Paris in 1835, homeopathy had established a strong foothold in medical practice. Homeopathy was introduced in France by Sebastien Maxime, Comte des Guidi, a nobleman and a refugee from Naples. He studied science and medicine at a college in Lyons and set up a homeopathic practice in Lyons in 1830, after an Italian homeopathic physician, Dr. de Romani, cured his wife of a reputedly incurable disease. Dr. des Guidi rapidly began to attract disciples because of his success in healing and his writings. In 1833, the Homeopathic Congress of Lyons awarded him a medal, recognizing his work in establishing homeopathy in France. When Dr. des Guidi was presented to the Emperor Napoleon III on his visit to Lyons in 1860, the Empress Eugénie hailed his "great service to humanity."

The Gallic Homeopathic Society was formed in 1832, in spite of opposition from the French Academy of Medicine. On Hahnemann's arrival in Paris three years later, the Society organized a festival in his honor, at which its President, Dr. Leon Simon, gave a speech of welcome. The Society awarded Hahnemann an honorary diploma late in 1834 and played a prominent part in the organization of the ceremonies at the reinterment of Hahnemann's body in the Père Lachaise Cemetery in Paris in 1898.

Dr. Benoit Mure, another stalwart of homeopathy in France, was born in Lyons. The son of a silk merchant, he founded the Homeopathic Institute of France in Paris in 1839 and opened two dispensaries.

Another great homeopathic physician was Dr. Jean-Pierre Gallvardin, who qualified in medicine in 1854 after studying with Dr. des Guidi. After years of fighting the medical establishment, he finally established a homeopathic hospital in Lyons in 1878. It still exists today.

In 1855, Dr. Jean-Pierre Tessier, head of the Beaugon Hospital, wrote a review entitled "The Medical Art," strongly supporting homeopathy. Five years later, France had more than 400 homeopathic physicians and eleven homeopathic pharmacies, six of which were in Paris. Three homeopathic hospitals were established in quick succession, the last of these being the St. Jacques Hospital, established in 1878 by Dr. P. Jonsset, a student of Dr. Tessier. Dr. Jonsset laid the foundations of modern homeopathy in France.

Although homeopathy declined in France in the late 19th and early 20th centuries, it did not decline to the same extent as in other countries. Homeopathy has always enjoyed vigorous support, and France may now hold the distinction of being the world's leading country in homeopathy. In 1987, 20 percent of the French population received homeopathic treatment regularly and more than 30 percent occasionally. Over 8,500 physicians of a total of 80,000 nationally practice homeopathy, and 1,200 veterinarians practice some homeopathy.

In spite of opposition in the medical and scientific press, the French Government has officially recognized homeopathic medicine through its acceptance of the *French Pharmacopoeia*. The 8th edition of this *Pharmacopoeia* was published in 1965 and it was reedited in 1983. The cost of homeopathic treatment in France is reimbursed through the National Medical Insurance system, but it only represents 0.25 percent of its budget. The average cost of a homeopathic prescription is only one-third of the cost of an allopathic prescription.

As early as 1912, Dr. Leon Vannier set up a structured teaching program for homeopathic physicians. Presently, homeopathic physicians receive training at the French School of Homeopathy, the Homeopathic Center of Studies, the Boiron Institute and the Medical Society of Biotherapies. Veterinary homeopathy is taught under the aegis of the Society of Veterinary Homeopathy, which was established in 1983, at centers in Maison-Alfrt, Toulouse and Nantes. In 1976, the first university diploma in homeopathy was created in Lyons.

The principal professional organization for qualified homeopathic physicians is the National Center for Homeopathy, with its headquarters in Paris. Like the United States and Britain, there are many local homeopathic associations for lay people throughout the country which hold regular meetings and study groups.

A special feature of French homeopathy is that the most frequently prescribed potencies are 4CH, 5CH, 7CH, 9CH, 15CH and 30CH, in contrast to those most frequently prescribed in most other countries—6x, 12x, 30x, 6CH, 12CH and 30CH. Potencies above 30CH are not legally permitted in France.

The considerable progress of homeopathy in France owes much to the two principal manufacturers of homeopathic medicines—Boiron and Dolisos. The former company established central homeopathic laboratories in Ste. Foy-Les Lyon in 1974 and the latter company in Montrichard. Both laboratories have excellent modern facilities and are situated in unpolluted rural areas. Both Boiron and Dolisos are engaged in teaching activities and homeopathic research programs and have developed internationally. Homeopathic research is now being conducted, through the initiative of these companies, in many universities throughout France.

HOMEOPATHY IN INDIA

Homeopathy began in India in 1828, when Maharajah Rangitsingh was treated for facial paralysis with Dulcamara by Dr. Hornbinger in Calcutta.

In the early 1830s, homeopathic clinics were established in Bombay, Delhi, Calcutta and, since then, homeopathy has been vigorously supported in India. At its peak in 1900 there were 400,000 homeopathic practitioners in the country.

Until his death in 1948, Mahatma Gandhi relied solely on homeopathic treatment and often spoke publicly of its value. Soon after India gained its independence, however, Pandit Jawaharlal Nehru passed a resolution that allopathic medicine would be the official system and called for more research into homeopathy and the Indian system of medicine. This resolution was reversed, however, by Mrs. Indira Gandhi in 1968, when she called on all state governments to recognize homeopathy and to include its use in their health plans.

In 1962, Dr. K. G. Saxena was appointed the first Homeopathic Advisor to the Indian Government. He and his successors, in this part-time appointment, were advised for 13 years on homeopathic development by the National Homeopathic Advisory Committee. With the formation of the Central Council of Homeopathy in 1975, the Homeopathic Advisory Committee was abolished. The post of Homeopathic Advisor remains a part-time role, in spite of efforts to make it a full-time appointment.

In 1963, a Homeopathic Research Committee was established and the central government started giving grants on the recommendation of this committee. A composite Research Council was formed five years later, embracing both homeopathy and the

Indian system of medicine, but, in 1978, a separate Research Council for homeopathy was constituted by the central government. Today there are 46 research centers throughout the country.

The Indian Institute of Homeopathic Physicians (IIHP), the professional body for qualified physicians, holds the All India Homeopathic Congress every two years. The 12th Congress was held in Ranchi in 1986, and attracted more than 1,000 delegates. In his valedictory address, the Indian film star Shri Shatrughan Sinha appealed for state governments to utilize homeopathy in the service of poor people of India. The 1988 Congress was held in Lucknow.

There are now more than 100,000 homeopathic practitioners in India, of which about 25,000 are Doctors of Medicine. As in most other countries, homeopathy has enjoyed a substantial growth in India over the last ten years.

2 FUNDAMENTALS OF HOMEOPATHY

Samuel Hahnemann's basic medical philosophy was well expressed in his writings:

> The physician's high and only mission is to restore the sick to health, to cure as it is termed. The highest ideal of cure is rapid, gentle and permanent restoration of health; or removal and annihilation of the disease in its whole extent, in the shortest, most reliable, and most harmless way, on easily comprehensible principles.
>
> If the physician clearly perceives what is to be cured in diseases, if he clearly perceives what is curative in each medicine and if he knows how to adapt, according to clearly defined principles, what is curative in medicines to what he has discovered to be morbid in the patient—to adapt it as well in respect of suitability of medicines as also in respect of the proper dose and the proper period for repeating the dose: if, finally he knows the obstacles to recovery in each case and is aware how to remove them, so that the restoration may be permanent, then he understands how to treat judiciously and rationally, and he is a true practitioner of the healing art.

LAW OF SIMILARS

The word homeopathy was derived by Samuel Hahnemann from the Greek words *homoios*, meaning like or similar, and *pathos*, meaning suffering. Hence, "like suffering" encompasses the basic principle of homeopathy, that is, treating "like with like".*

---

*The Greek word *homoios* (similar) should not be confused with the word *homos* (same). Hahnemann often expressed his annoyance when allopaths referred to his new therapy as Homopathy.

Hahnemann asserted the truth of the principle with the Latin phrase

Similia similibus curentur
"Let likes be treated by likes"

Hahnemann expressed it thus:
"Every medicine which, among the symptoms it can cause in a healthy body, reproduces those most present in a given disease, capable of curing that disease in the swiftest, most thorough and most enduring fashion."

This is known as the simile principle, or the Law of Similars. By this principle a homeopathic remedy is selected for its ability to produce similar symptoms in a healthy person to those experienced by the patient.

Following his epoch-making experiment with Cinchona when translating Cullen's *Materia Medica* in 1790, Hahnemann proceeded to test the effects of large doses of plant extracts on himself, carefully noting the symptoms they produced. The results of these *provings* were published in his book, *Fragmenta de Viribus Medicamentorum Positivus Sive in San Corpore Humano Observatis.* The first part of the book listed the symptoms produced by substances on the human body and the second part listed 26 homeopathic remedies, including Arnica Montana, Atropa Belladonna, Chamomilla, Ignatia Amara, Pulsatilla Nigricans and Rhus Toxicodendron.

Subsequently, Hahnemann recruited a group of collaborators to assist him in the systematic proving of a new range of medicines. He laid down strict procedures to ensure accuracy. The prover was required to write down the time of each dose, note every symptom and the time of its onset, and so on. In addition, the prover was required to abstain from alcohol and tea or coffee and keep to a regular diet.

The results of these provings were published in Hahnemann's *Materia Medica Pura* in which several thousand symptoms were recorded for 66 individual medicines.

Hahnemann wrote:

> On every occasion when my Leipzig colleagues delivered their reports on provings, I questioned them in respect of the symptoms they had observed in order to get as precisely as possible the verbal expressions of their sensations and sufferings, and to ascertain exactly the conditions under which the symptoms occurred. I also checked that they

had observed the carefully regulated diet during their provings.

The range of symptoms which any substance can cause is called the *drug picture*. The totality of symptoms of a particular disease is called the *disease picture*. The homeopathic approach, therefore, is to match these pictures as closely as possible to achieve the best therapeutic results. For example, Atropa Belladonna (or Deadly Nightshade), given to a healthy person would induce *inter alia*, a flushed face and a high fever. The prime symptoms of scarlet fever are a flushed face and a high fever. Atropa Belladonna in homeopathic doses is, therefore, an appropriate treatment for scarlet fever. As another example, Ipecacuanha, in large doses, induces nausea and vomiting, whereas in minute potentized homeopathic doses, it is a treatment for nausea and vomiting. This may be seen as an inversion of pharmacological activity.

The symptoms experienced by the patient—both physical and mental—are of great importance in homeopathy. Only by building up a detailed symptom picture can the "similimum" be found. Although the symptoms of most diseases are more or less clearly defined, a closer study of individual patients shows variations from one to another. Each person is unique and, in treating the whole person, different homeopathic medicines may be required to treat different people suffering from the same disease.

The conventional view is that symptoms are a direct manifestation of a disease, whereas the homeopathic view is that the symptoms are a manifestation of the body's fight, by its natural defense mechanism, to overcome the disease. Homeopathy, therefore, seeks to stimulate these symptoms, however briefly, and not to suppress them. In stimulating the symptoms, homeopathic medicine is seen to assist the body's natural forces for recovery.

A brief or transient worsening of the patient's symptoms resulting from a homeopathic dose is not unusual in chronic cases. Such a reaction is called the *homeopathic aggravation* and is an indication that the medicine is taking effect. The increase in the severity of the symptoms may be very slight and be of a few seconds duration and barely noticeable. If the increase in severity is marked or prolonged, the patient is said to be proving the medicine. The sign < is used to denote an aggravation. In practice, Hahnemann found that the aggravation was maintained with smaller doses (potencies) of the medicines.

The diagram below is a simplified illustration of the homeopathic approach to illness in contrast to allopathy.

HERING'S LAW

Dr. Constantine Hering provided useful guidance in monitoring
the progress of homeopathic treatment with respect to symptoms. This law states that symptoms improve during homeopathic treatment from above downwards, from the most vital to
the least vital organ and from the latest to the earliest symptoms.

POSOLOGY

The Infinitesimal Dose

Hahnemann had long held the conviction that medicines
should be prescribed in small doses. As early as 1788, more than

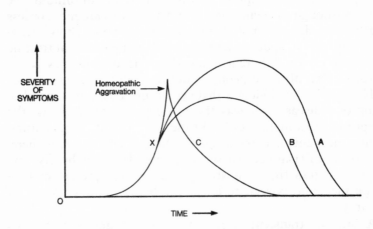

Curve A represents the course of a disease when left
untreated. The symptoms increase to maximum severity and then decrease as the natural healing forces overcome the disease. Curve B represents allopathic treatment started after the onset of the disease at X. The
symptoms are suppressed and peak out at a lower
severity with less discomfort for the patient. Curve C
represents homeopathic treatment started after the onset of the disease at X. The homeopathic aggravation
temporarily worsens the symptoms, then is followed
by a complete and effective cure.

twenty years before the publication of his *Organon*, his article, "An Unusually Strong Remedy for Checking Putrefaction," advised the use of a solution of only one part silver nitrate in 1,000 parts of water.

In his *Organon* he advanced his doctrine of the minimum dose: "The *very smallest doses* of medicine chosen for the homeopathic diseases are each a match for the corresponding disorders. The physician will choose a homeopathic remedy in just *so small a dose* as will overcome the disease."

His original aim was to determine the smallest effective dose in order to minimize any poisonous side effects and make the treatment as safe as possible. He found, however, that on progressively diluting the medicines, not only did they retain their effectiveness, but for certain conditions they were more efficacious.

Hahnemann developed a precise, scientific method of serial or sequential dilution of the *mother tinctures* he had prepared from therapeutic substances, in alcohol/water solutions. The serial dilutions were carried out in ratios of 1:10 (decimal series) and 1:100 (centesimal series). Each dilution, or attenuation, was followed by the process of succussion, or dynamization, to produce homeopathic *potencies* (See Chapter 3). He described the method as potentization.

Thus, even for a relatively low potency such as 6x, diluted and dynamized six times in the prescribed matter, is a dilution of one part of the mother tincture in one million parts of alcohol/water mixture (1×10^6). The quantity of active ingredient in this dilution is much less than even the lowest allopathic dose. For example, a low allopathic dose of one milligram is in the order of 1,000 times a homeopathic potency of 6x. An intermediate potency, such as 30CH, represents an infinitesimally small dose of one part of the mother tincture of 10^{60} parts of alcohol/water mixture.

Hahnemann wrote, in 1838; on the nature of potencies:

> "Homeopathic dynamizations are processes by which the decimal properties, which are latent in natural substances, while in their crude state, become aroused and then become enabled to act in an almost spiritual manner on our life, that is on our sensible and irritable fiber. These preparations cannot simply be designated as dilutions, although every preparation of this kind, in order that it may be raised to a higher potency (that is, in order for the intrinsic properties still latent within it to be

further awakened and developed) must first undergo a further attenuation in order that the trituration of succusion may enter still further into
the very essence of the medicinal substances and
may thus also liberate and expose the more subtle part of the medicinal powers hidden deeply,
which could not be effected by trituration and
succusions in the concentrated form.

Potencies of insoluble substances are prepared by the process
of trituration (see Chapter 3) in their solid form.

The minute doses of homeopathic potencies are believed to
act as a catalyst to stimulate the body's natural defense mechanism to combat the disease. If this is the case, it follows, therefore, that the homeopathic medicine itself acts indirectly in
effecting the cure. It is now accepted, by allopaths and homeopaths alike, that the body's curative mechanism involves the
production of only minute quantities of complex chemical substances within the body to counter the invasion of disease viruses (See Chapter 5).

Arndt-Schultz Law

The Arndt-Schultz law with reference to biological activity
provides justification for the use of minute doses. This law
states that small doses of drugs encourage life activity, large
material doses of drugs impede life activity and very large doses
destroy life activity. To put it another way, the function of the
dose of the drug is inversely proportional to the effect of the
drug.

The posological concept of the infinitesimally small dose is
the second basic principle of homeopathy. Apart from their therapeutic effectiveness, minute homeopathic dosages render even
the most toxic substances used in their preparation safe and free
from unwanted side effects.

It is a basic tenet of homeopathy, as a natural therapy, that
the medicines are derived from natural sources, whether these
sources be plant, mineral, animal or biological. Synthesized
chemicals are rarely used in homeopathy, which relies on the
synergistic complexity of natural substances. Each homeopathic
medicine has its own essence and vitality, through a subtle
blend of substances found only in nature.

The pharmacology of these medicines reveals affinities for
certain glands, organs or tissues, which suggests their possible

use. Similarly, many homeopathic medicines are closely related to the physical, mental and emotional characteristics of the patient, and this again influences their use. From these considerations, we can derive the homeopathic *drug picture*, which must be matched with the patient.

Although the pharmaceutical forms of homeopathic medicines and their modes of administration to the patient are identical with allopathic medicines, their preparation and the manner in which they are prescribed are quite different.

TREATING THE WHOLE PERSON

Homeopathy is truly a holistic medical practice in that it treats the whole person. It recognizes that every person is unique. As Dr. Margery Blackie wrote, the homeopathic physician concentrates on the patient, not the cure. Because every patient is different, the physician does not always prescribe a specific medicine for a specific disease, but prescribes on an individual basis.

Again quoting Hahnemann, in his *The Chronic Diseases: their Peculiar Nature and their Homopathic Cure* (1828): "The physician's first duty is to enquire into the whole condition of the patient: the cause of the disease, his or her mode of life, the nature of his or her mind, the tone or character of his or her sentiments, his or her physical constitution and then especially, the symptoms of the disease."

Factors which cause an illness are of prime importance in the homeopathic system, since they enable us to optimize the individualistic approach to treatment. People react differently to factors which cause an illness, such as infection, emotional stress, lifestyle or diet, depending on their hereditary, physical and psychological patterns.

In his later years, Hahnemann turned from science and medicine to philosophy and attempted to explain the true nature of disease and the fundamental mechanism of homeopathy. His book, *The Chronic Diseases*, announced his discovery of the cause of chronic disease—the theory of *miasms*. He believed the miasm to be an agent that was passed down from generation to generation, a hereditary mechanism that acted within the body. In this theory he was progressing beyond the strict application of the Law of Similars. Nowadays, we would study the miasm theory in terms of our knowledge of the genetic code and the existence of DNA (deoxyribonucleic acid) and RNA (ribonucleic acid), which we know play an important part in hereditary characteristics.

Hahnemann defined three diatheses, when groups of individuals presented analogous symptoms in their illnesses through hereditary factors. These are:

1. *Sycosis* Resulting from attacks on the genito-urinary system.
2. *Syphilis (Luetism)* Resulting from syphilis in previous generations.
3. *Psora* A range of diseases, not included in the first two diatheses, related to the skin.

In recent years, the AIDS (Acquired Immune Deficiency Syndrome) epidemic has focused attention on the reduction or destruction of the immune system, thus impairing the body's natural defense mechanisms. Research has concentrated on the development of an AIDS vaccine or antiviral treatment, but the homeopathic approach would be to improve the effectiveness of the body's natural defenses.

A disease can establish itself in the body when the efficiency of the immune system is impaired. Viruses in the body, passed down from generation to generation in a dormant state, can become active when the efficiency of the immune system is lowered. Poor physical and mental condition encourages these viruses to become active. Infections particularly susceptible to this phenomenon include herpes, shingles and viral pneumonia.

The origin of the illness is usually related to a specific event, such as an accident. They may include muscle or back strain through overexertion, exposure or heart strain.

Any mental attitude which is contrary to a person's harmony with nature can lower his or her immunity. Tension, fear, stress and anxiety have an enormous capacity to alter the chemistry of the body. This is particularly relevant in our modern stressful society, with its overcrowding, competitiveness, fast-moving technological advances, fear of a nuclear holocaust, drug and sexual problems, to mention only a few.

The psychological state of the patient is, therefore, of great importance to the homeopathic physician in deciding the treatment. Many illnesses are the direct result of the wrong lifestyle with all the excesses of the patient. Conventional medicine is often concerned not with curing the disease, but with suppressing the severity of the symptoms to a level that enables patients to continue "instantly" the habits and lifestyle with which they wish to persevere. The patient is thus caught in a vicious circle.

Hahnemann believed that homeopathic treatment must be coupled with adequate sleep, exercise and proper diet to effect a complete and permanent cure. The patients who benefit most from homeopathic treatment are those who, with the assistance of a physician, are prepared to improve the quality of their lives by avoiding excesses, eradicating areas of their lives which depress and agitate, bringing forth their suppressed emotions and, not the least important, indulging in laughter and happiness. The removal of these stresses, together with the appropriate homeopathic medicine will stimulate the body's defense mechanism.

Specific examples of psychological causes and specific treatments are grief—Ignatia; mental strain—Acidum Phosphoricum or Kalium Phosphoricum; fear—Aconitum Napellus.

THE HOLISTIC APPROACH OF HOMEOPATHY

Hahnemann, always ahead of his time, perceived the need to treat the whole person and not simply the disease. In seeking an explanation of the holistic approach to medicine, we may ask whether the whole person is more than the sum of his or her parts. The fragmented approach identifies the parts, how they operate, why they fail and how to cure them; this reductionist approach has proved its usefulness, (F. Capra, 1982).

Although the quality of the individual parts must influence the illness, the biochemical model cannot take into account the social, psychological and environmental context in which the parts function, how the person thinks, behaves and relates to others, or how lifestyle influences the ways the parts operate. We should replace the mechanistic approach to the study of health and disease with a humanistic approach, where sharing, caring, loving, touching and hoping play as important a role in our endeavors as the study of pathology and biochemistry (P. Pietroni, 1984).

The whole person is acknowledged to be multidimensional, responding to and developing within a social and environmental context. Mind and nature form a necessary unity (G. Bateson, 1979). Research indicates that feelings and experiences change us even at cellular level. Mind and body constantly interact and influence one another. Physicians, therefore, must be concerned with biological, psychological and sociological factors, since holistic medicine accepts that all these systems influence one another—change one and you change them all (G. Engel, 1977). Additionally, we must consider how the patient relates to past experiences, the present and the future and how he or she adapts to them.

Homeopathy recognizes that patients are rarely passive recipients of their treatment. Self-help and prevention are intrinsic to homeopathy. Patients must be involved with their treatment and accept that changes in their lifestyle, diet, habits, philosophy, control of stress and the sheer willpower to regain their health are interrelated. K. Pelletier (1978) affirms that the negative effects of the reluctant patient can be overcome. In these ways the natural healing forces within the body are optimized. The adage, "Physician Heal Thyself," is appropriate to homeopathy, since the physician needs to develop the potential for caring, responsiveness and adaptability before he or she is able to help others (Holistic Medicine, 1988). The patient needs the kindness, sympathy, patience, tolerance, understanding and empathy of the physician or practitioner. Neither can spiritual factors be wholly ignored. Treatment cannot be by medicine alone, as healing is the result of making people whole.

MODALITIES

Modalities are defined as influences which worsen (aggravation) or improve (amelioration) the symptoms of the patient. These influences are an invaluable guide to the choice of a homeopathic remedy. Modalities are manifested in several forms, which are grouped as follows:

(1) Physical Modalities

These modalities are associated with movement, position of body (e.g., lying down or sitting), touch, rest, exertion, effects of light, noise and smells.

(2) Temperature Modalities

A most important modality is related to the effect of cold and warmth on the patient. This includes the effect of cold wind and other climatic factors, such as damp and seasons of the year.

(3) Time Modalities

Time modalities involve the improvement or worsening of the symptoms during periods of the day or at precise times.

(a) Day or night
(b) Morning, afternoon or evening
(c) Hourly, e.g., 10 a.m. or 1 a.m. to 3 a.m.

(4) Dietary Modalities

Modalities induced by certain foods or types of food and drinks, including alcohol. Likes and dislikes of particular foods and drinks are also relevant.

(5) Localized Modalities (Lateralities)

Just as there are left-handed and right-handed people, so do we have modalities which affect the left side or the right side of the body. Many homeopathic remedies are particularly suited to left side or the right side. For example, neuralgia on the right side of the face indicates Atropa Belladonna. The modality may alternate between left and right. From left to right, Lachesis is indicated, and from right to left, Lycopodium is indicated. Details of modalities are given in subsequent chapters.

The success of homeopathic treatment, therefore, relies upon the skillful application of the Law of Similars, the study of the patient as a whole person—physically and psychologically—causal factors and modalities and the administration of the appropriate medicine in the correct potency.

MATERIA MEDICA AND REPERTORY

Although there are many useful textbooks on homeopathy, the fundamental reference works are the *Homeopathic Materia Medicas* and *Repertories*. In these *Materia Medicas*, homeopathic remedies are listed in alphabetical order. The symptoms relating to each homeopathic remedy are listed logically under the headings of different anatomical sections in which they have occurred or in a general section. *Materia Medicas* were the original provings of the remedies and from clinical experience and include, *Materia Medica Pura* (Samuel Hahnemann); *Materia*

Medica with Repertory (W. Boericke); *Repertory of Homeopathic Materia Medica* (J.T. Kent); *Guiding Symptoms* (C. Hering); and the *Dictionary of Practical Materia Medica* (J.H. Clark). (See Chapter 4.)

There is no substitute for the constant, day-to-day use of the *Materia Medica* in homeopathic practice. After taking a case history, noting the most important symptoms together with their causalities and modalities, reference is made to the *Materia Medica* in the appropriate anatomical, general or mind sections to select the remedy most strongly indicated as suitable for the needs of the patient.

In recent times, much of the information given in the *Materia Medica* is available in computer data-banks, enabling a swift and accurate choice of the appropriate remedy.

APPLIED HOMEOPATHY

Other important fields of homeopathy, which may be described collectively as *applied homeopathy*, are discussed in subsequent chapters. Applied homeopathy may be defined broadly as the application of more than one remedy at the same time, or single remedies which do not have a full drug picture given in the *Materia Medica* and, as such, have more specific uses.

This branch of homeopathy includes Isodes (from the patient); Nosodes (diseased tissue, with limited symptom picture); Allergens, Combination Remedies (polypharmacy); and the Biotherapies which embrace Organotherapy (sarcodes—healthy organs, glands or tissues from animals); Gemmotherapy (buds or young shoots of plants); and Dechelating Lithotherapy (mineral ores).

HOMEOPATHICALLY-RELATED THERAPIES

Biochemic Remedies

These remedies are also known as *Schüssler Salts, Cell Salts* or *Tissue Salts*. They are based on a system of medicine introduced by a German physician, Dr. Schüssler, who originally practiced homeopathy. The theory of this system is based on the observation that all diseases are related to a deficiency of mineral salts in the body, which bears no relation to the homeopathic principles, but is loosely related to Dechelating Lithotherapy. (See Chapter 5.)

The Biochemic Remedies, however, are prepared homeopathically as triturated, compressed tablets (see Chapter 3) in 6x potency.

The twelve remedies are:

Calcarea Carbonica 6x	Kalium Phosphoricum 6x
Calcarea Fluorica 6x	Kalium Muriaticum 6x
Calcarea Phosphorica 6x	Kalium Sulphuricum 6x
Calcarea Sulphuricum 6x	Natrum Muriaticum 6x
Ferrous Phosphoricum 6x	Natrum Phosphoricum 6x
Magnesia Phosphorica 6x	Silica 6x

Bach Remedies

These remedies are not homeopathic, since they are not prepared in potencies, but they are considered by many to be analogous to homeopathic remedies.

Introduced by Dr. Edward Bach in England in the early 1930s, they comprise 38 remedies prepared from fresh flowers, trees and special waters. Each remedy is associated with a specific set of emotional experiences. The basis of Dr. Bach's theory was that all diseases are of mental origin and they are, therefore, prescribed on the basis of the mental indications of the patient only. Examples of Bach remedies are Rock Rose (fear) and Mimulus (shock).

A special Bach (pronounced "batch") remedy is called the Rescue Remedy, indicated for treatment in emergencies. It actually consists of five Remedies: Star of Bethlehem (shock); Rock Rose (panic and terror); Impatiens (tension and mental stress); Cherry Plum (desperation); and Clematis (fainting or loss of consciousness).

Veterinary Homeopathy

Homeopathy is particularly effective in the treatment of babies and young children and, in recent years, veterinary homeopathy has taken a great leap forward. The success of homeopathic medicine in these fields counters its critics, who claim that homeopathic cure is entirely psychosomatic.

HOMEOPATHY AND ALLOPATHY

Homeopaths recognize that surgery is sometimes essential, although in some cases homeopathic treatment can bring about a cure, for example, for stomach ulcers. Homeopathic medicines can also assist in postoperative recovery. Antibiotics would also be recommended for severe infections, as would the conventional treatment of the body's deficiencies, such as iron, vitamin or trace element deficiencies. In the latter case, however, dechelating lithotherapy may be appropriate (See Chapter 5).

Paracelsus held strong views on what was required in a successful physician. "Like each plant and metallic remedy," he wrote, "the doctor too must have a specific virtue. He must be intimate with Nature. He must have the intuition which is necessary to understand the patient, his body, his disease. He must have the feel and touch which makes it possible for him to be in sympathetic communication with the patient's spirits." He believed that the success of the physician depends to a great extent on his ability to give the patient confidence and mobilize his will to health.

Dr. Glin Bennet (The Wound and the Doctor, 1987) suggested that allopathic physicians are entrapped within a model of medicine which is mechanistic, preoccupied with authority, rewards a tough-minded attitude toward people and their feelings. Modern medicine exacts a fierce price from both patient and doctor in that it disregards their humanity, frailty and feelings and exaggerates their similarity with machines. Doctors, he argued, should take into account not only the body but also the mind and spirit as well, and encourage patients to mobilize whatever healing potential they possess within themselves and exploit their own limitations and vulnerability in forming therapeutic relationship with patients.

Whether he knew it or not, Dr. Bennet was expressing the homeopathic philosophy of cure and the relationship between the patient and the doctor. For therein lies the key to its successful and rewarding practice. The disposition of the homeopathic practitioner ranks in importance with the fundamental truth of homeopathy.

Homeopathy is natural, safe and compassionate therapy which relies on its fundamental precepts, the attitude and utmost skill of the practitioner and the patience and cooperation of the patient. It is not a panacea for all ills, offering instant cure for every illness, but more a way of life. It stands on its impressive track record of almost 200 years in the relief of suffering.

3 HOMEOPATHIC PHARMACY

Homeopathic preparations may be described as medicaments prepared in accordance with the methods described in the *Homeopathic Materia Medica* and the latest edition of the British, French or American *Homeopathic Pharmacopoeia*. The last British edition was published at the end of the last century, but the Review Committee of the *Homeopathic Pharmacopoeia of the United States* is planning to publish the 9th Edition in 1989. The *Pharmacopoeia* sets out the approved procedures for the preparation of the medicines. In the series of monographs, the sources of the medicaments are listed alphabetically, including their proper "generic" names, common names, formulae where appropriate, descriptions of the sources, minimum potencies recommended for prescriptions and over-the-counter supply, references and technical data.

CLASSIFICATION OF HOMEOPATHIC MEDICINES

There are more than 3,000 homeopathic medicines. They may be classified in two ways—according to the origin or source of the medicine or in the manner in which they are prescribed.

1. *Sources* a) Plant vegetable substances
b) Animal substances
c) Chemical elements and minerals
d) Biological sources

2. *Methods* a) Specific remedies
of Application b) Polychrest remedies
c) Constitutional remedies
d) Combination remedies
e) Single remedies

In this chapter only the "Sources" are relevant. The second category is discussed in a subsequent chapter.

Plant Substances

More than 60 percent of all remedies are derived from plant substances, which include whole plants, flowers, leaves, stems, bark, woods, roots, buds, berries, fruits, seeds, bulbs or corms.

Plant specimens are collected in their natural habitats or grown organically—without the application of pesticides or artificial fertilizers—in special nurseries or recognized botanical gardens.

Whole Plants

The fresh, succulent plants are collected in the flowering season in sunny weather. They are cleaned by gentle shaking in hot water to remove dirt, insects, etc. Examples are:

Aconitum Napellus (Aconite, Monkshood, Wolfsbane). Tall plant with flowers shaped like a monk's cowl; grows in mountainous areas.

Calendula Officinalis (Common Marigold). Sometimes the roots are excluded.

Chamomilla (Wild Chamomile). An annual herb growing in Europe, Northern Asia and India. One of the original remedies proved by Samuel Hahnemann.

Leaves

Leaves are collected when fully developed, shortly before the flowering season or after sunset. Example:

Rhus Toxicodendron (Rhus Tox., Poison Ivy). Very poisonous shrub growing in the United States.

Flowers

Collected in dry weather, just as they are beginning to open. Flowers alone are rarely used.

Roots

Roots of annual plants are best lifted after the seeds have ripened in the early Fall. Biennials are best lifted in the Spring and perennials in the second or third year. They must be washed thoroughly and carefully inspected for signs of mold growth or woody appearance. Examples are:

Ipecacuanha (Ipecac). Contains several alkaloids, mainly emetine.

Bryonia Alba (White Bryony, Wild Hops). Climbing hedgerow plant, growing in Europe. One of the original remedies proved by Samuel Hahnemann.

Bryonia Dioica has a similar therapeutic action.

Barks

Non-resinous barks are collected from young trees in the late autumn. Barks from resinous trees are collected during the development of blossom and leaves. Example:

Cinchona (China, Peruvian Bark). The bark of the quinaquina tree has a high quinine content. Indigenous to South America. Used by Samuel Hahnemann in his original proving experiment.

Berries, Fruits and Seeds

Perfect specimens, gathered when ripe, with only a few exceptions. Dried seeds may be stored in a closed container in a cool place in laboratories. They are inspected for moldiness, bad smell or discoloration. Examples are:

Nux Vomica (Nux Vom., Poison Nut). Dried seeds from the orange berries of a tree with crooked trunk, growing in Northern Australia. The seeds contain several aklaloids, mainly strychnine, and are very poisonous.

Phytolacca Decandra (Phytolacca, Virginian Poke). Tall herbaceous plant with clusters of purple/black berries and greenish/ pink flowers. Native plant of America. The whole plant, including the berries, is used to prepare the remedy.

Ignatia Amara (Ignatia, St. Ignatius Bean). Prepared from the seeds of the plant, which is indigenous to the Philippines.

Bulbs and Corms

Bulbs and corms are lifted from the soil in March or April. Example:

Colchicum Autumnale (Colchicum, Autumn crocus). Large corm, about 3.5 centimeters in diameter, with white or pale rose flower, growing in damp meadows. The main constituent is the alkaloid, colchicine.

Buds and Shoots

Buds and young shoots of plants, trees and shrubs are rich in growth factors, including hormones, auxins and gibberellins. These remedies belong to a branch of homeopathy known as Gemmotherapy, developed in France. Gemmotherapy is discussed in Chapter 5, pages 111–112. Examples:

Ribes Nigrum, (Black Currant). Prepared from glycerine macerates fresh buds, which are rich in vitamin C, anthocyanins and flavonoids and possess antiinflammatory properties.

Pinus Montana (Mountain Pine). Prepared from glycerine macerates fresh buds of the tree, which have an entrophic effect of the articular cartilage.

Animal Substances

These substances, which may be parts of, or whole animals, are obtained only from perfect, healthy specimens. They are collected in the wild or from zoos. Animal sources of homeopathic remedies are the second largest group, accounting for about 20 percent of the remedies. They must not be mixed with other substances and they should be stored in well-sealed containers in a cool, dark place. Some examples are as follows:

Apis Mellifica (Apis Mel., Honey Bee). Prepared from the fresh whole bee.

Cantharis (Spanish fly, Blister Beetle). A small, brilliant blue-green beetle about 2 centimeters in length, with a strong odor. The dried, powdered insect is used.

Sepia Officinalis (Sepia, Cuttlefish juice). Prepared from the brown, inky juice exuded by the cuttlefish on the approach of a predator.

Lachesis mutus (Lachesis, Bushmaster Snake, Surukuku). Prepared from the poisonous venom of the Bushmaster snake. The original proving was carried out by Dr. Constantine Hering during his travels in South America.

Tarantula Hispanica (Tarantula Hisp., Spanish Spider, Lycosa Tarantula). A bite from this poisonous spider was thought to cause hysteria for which dancing was the cure, hence *tarantella*.

Chemical Elements and Minerals

Sources of medicines in this category are subdivided into those substances which are soluble in alcohol or water, and those which are insoluble. Mother tinctures of insoluble elements and minerals are prepared by trituration, a technique discussed later in this chapter.

Where possible, minerals from naturally occurring ores are used rather than synthetic. Substances may be organic or inorganic compounds. Some examples are as follows:

Arsenicum Album (Arsen Alb., Arseneous oxide). Insoluble, white powder, Formula As_2O_3.

Carbo Vegetabilis (Vegetable Charcoal). The residue from the controlled burning of beech or birch wood. Amorphous (that is, no regular shape) black carbon with traces of several mineral salts. Insoluble in alcohol/water.

Hepar Sulphuris (Calcium Sulfide). One of the original remedies proved by Samuel Hahnemann. Prepared by heating equal parts of finely powdered oyster shell (Calcium Carbonate) and pure sulfur to white heat. Formula: CaS. Insoluble in alcohol/water.

Kalium Bichromicum (Kali Bich., Potassium Bichromate, Potassium Dichromate). An orange-red crystalline salt prepared from naturally occurring chromium ore with the formula $K_2Cr_2O_7$ in its anhydrous form.

Natrum Muriaticum (Nat Mur., Sodium Chloride, Common Salt). Prepared from naturally occurring rock salt as white crystals or powder. Formula: NaCl.

Plumbum Metallicum (Plumbum Met., Lead Metal). Symbol Pb. Bluish-white, grey metal extracted from the naturally occurring ore, galena (Lead Sulphide). Insoluble in alcohol/water.

Silica (Silica, Silicon Dioxide). White powder or transparent crystals with the formula SiO_2. Occurs naturally as flint, quartz, agate and sand. Insoluble in alcohol/water.

Calcarea Carbonica (Calc. Carb., Calcium Carbonate, Formula: $CaCO_3$). Hahnemann used the soft, middle layer of the oyster shell as his source for this compound, which contains small quantities of impurities, such as magnesium carbonate and sodium chloride. Like many sources of homeopathic medicines, it is believed that this natural blend of compounds occurring in nature is superior to a single, pure synthesizied compound.

Biological Sources

There are two categories of these specialized homeopathic medicines. Fresh organs, glandular or tissue extracts removed from healthy pigs, sheep or cattle, called *sarcodes*, and morbid or diseased tissues (for example pus), called *nosodes*. The former extracts, using healthy specimens, belong to the branch of homeopathy called Organotherapy, developed in France, and will be discussed in a later chapter.

The bowel nosodes are a special type of nosode developed by Glasgow physicians Dr. John Paterson and Dr. Edward Bach. These medicines are derived from cultures of stools containing intestinal bacteria. Examples are as follows:

Sarcodes: Adrenal gland, pancreas, kidney.

Nosodes: Influenzinum, Medorrhinum, Variolinum.

PREPARATION OF MOTHER TINCTURES

"Mother Tinctures" can be defined as the homeopathic medicament in its most concentrated form. They are produced as clear liquids or in solid triturated form. The liquids range from colorless to straw colored to dark brown or a red color. All mother tinctures are denoted by the Greek letter ɸ, or the abbreviation MT.

Mother tinctures of plant, vegetable or animal substances are prepared by the maceration of the fresh material in different strengths of alcohol at ambient temperature. After aging for periods ranging from one hour to one month, the suspension is filtered by gravity or compression. Final alcohol strengths may be 33⅓%, 50% or 80 to 90% (volume/volume), depending on the water content of the starting material.

Succulent, fresh plants yield between 350 to 700 ml of unfiltered succus (or juice) per kilogram of plant material. The succus is mixed with one half of its volume of 95% pure alcohol, producing mother tinctures of approximately 33⅓% (volume/volume) alcohol content.

Fresh plant material yielding less than 350 ml per kilogram of succus is repeatedly macerated with alcohol/water mixtures, producing mother tinctures of approximately 80 to 87% (volume/volume) alcohol content.

Mother tinctures for organotherapy preparations are prepared from macerates of buds or young shoots with alcoholized glycerin.

If properly stored, mother tinctures have an indefinite therapeutic activity, although it is sometimes necessary to remove precipitated solid matter by filtration from time to time.

PREPARATION OF POTENCIES

1. Hahnemann Methods

By systematic experimentation, Samuel Hahnemann determined that, by progressively diluting the mother tinctures to reduce the quantity of drug administered, he could not only render the treatment safe from all poisonous side effects, but also enhance the therapeutic activity—or make it stronger or more potent. He named these dilutions *potencies* and laid down a strict procedure. Hahnemann developed his method over many years and it was published in detail in the 4th edition of the *Organon*. He wrote: "Whenever a dilution of any kind is to be made, the name and number of the remedy are recorded on the labels of the appropriate number of flasks needed. These are then arranged one after the other. (see diagram).

"After introducing 99 drops of alcohol, one drop of the medicine undergoing dilution is poured from the first flask into the next. Always be sure that the drop taken from one flask is instilled in the next flask in line. The flask is then stoppered and shaken twice."

Potentization is carried out successively in two distinct steps—*dilution* and *succussion*. Thus, the process involves the sequential or serial dilution of the mother tincture with a mixture of alcohol and water. Each dilution is followed by succussion, which involves vigorous shaking with impact.

There are a series of dilutions: *decimal series*, based on serial dilutions of 1:10; *centesimal series*, based on serial dilutions of 1:100, and the *millesimal series*, based on serial dilutions of 1:1,000. Hence the decimal series of potencies is denoted 1x, 2x, 3x, 4x, . . . Nx, the centesimal series is denoted 1c, 2c, 3c, 4c, . . . Nc (denoted 1, 2, 3, 4, in the United Kingdom), and the millesimal series is denoted with the suffix m.

See page 55 for detailed treatment of potency nomenclature.

a) Decimal Potencies

The method of preparation is as follows:

To one part (or 1 ml) of mother tincture in a glass container is added 9 parts (or 9 ml) of alcohol/water and the mixture is succussed, giving a potency of 1x.

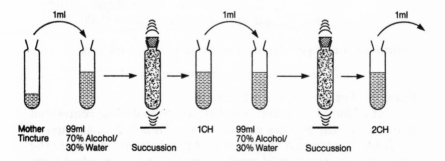

Mother Tincture | 99ml 70% Alcohol/ 30% Water | Succussion | 1CH | 99ml 70% Alcohol/ 30% Water | Succussion | 2CH

Diagram of Hahnemann Method of Potentization (Centesimal Series)

To one part (or 1ml) of a solution of potency 1x is added a further 9 parts (or 9 ml) of alcohol/water and the mixture is succussed again, giving a potency of 2x.

The serial dilution and succussion is repeated to produce progressively potencies of 3x, 4x, 5x, and so on up the series.

Thus, we have decimal dilutions as follows:

1x	1 part in 10	1:10	10^{-1}
2x	1 part in 100	1:1000	10^{-2}
3x	1 part in 1,000	1:1,000	10^{-3}
4x	1 part in 10,000	1:10,000	10^{-4}

Dilutions of any potency may be determined as follows:

$$Nx \ (N = \text{any potency number}) = 10^{-N}$$

Example: Let $N = 30$. Then $30x = 10^{-30}$

b) Centesimal Series

The method of preparation is as follows:

To one part (or 1 ml) of mother tincture in a glass container is added 99 parts (or 99 ml) of alcohol/water and the mixture is succussed, giving a potency of 1c.

To one part (or 1 ml) of a solution of potency 1c is added a further 99 parts (or 99 ml) of alcohol/water and the mixture is succussed again, giving a potency of 2c.

The progress is repeated to produce progressively potencies of 3c, 4c, 5c, and so on.

Thus we have centesimal dilutions as follows:

1c	1 part in 100	1:100	10^{-2}
2c	1 part in 10,000	1:10,000	10^{-4}
3c	1 part in 1,000,000	1:1,000,000	10^{-6}
4c	1 part in 100,000,000	1:100,000,000	10^{-8}

Dilutions of any potency may be determined as follows:

$$Nc \ (N = \text{any potency number}) = 10^{-24}$$

Example: Let $N = 12$. Then $12c = 10^{-24}$

In the United Kingdom it is customary to denote centesimal potencies by the potency number alone. Thus 1, 2, 3, 4, 5 and so on. It can be seen that the dilution of potencies 1c and 2x are the same, that is, one part of mother tincture in one hundred parts $(1:10^2)$ of alcohol/water.

Similarly:

2c is the same dilution as 4x $(1:10^4)$
3c is the same dilution as 6x $(1:10^6)$
4c is the same dilution as 8x $(1:10^8)$

However, it is incorrect to define potencies in terms of dilution alone, as, although dilution may be the same, the number of succussions which are an integral part of the potentization process are different. For example, the dilution of potencies of 3c and 6x are the same, but the former has required three dilutions and succussions and the latter six dilutions and succussions.

c) Millesimal series

A third potency series is the millesimal scale, based on dilutions of 1:1,000, which is rarely prescribed. In preparing millesimal potencies, the same procedure is employed as far as decimal and centesimal potencies, except that one part (or 1 ml of mother tincture is diluted sequentially with 999 parts (or 999 ml) of alcohol/water.

Potencies on the millesimal scale are sometimes denoted 1M, 2M, 3M etc., but this leads to confusion with the use of 1M to denote a centesimal potency of 1,000, as previously described. Another system, which is probably more explanatory, is to denote millesimal potencies by the suffix m.

It follows that millesimal dilutions are:

1m	1:1,000	10^{-3}
2m	1:1,000,000	10^{-6}
3m	1:1,000,000,000	10^{-9}
etc.		

2. Korsakovian Method

The Hahnemann method of dilution is both scientific and accurate and is, therefore, wholly acceptable. It remains the classic method to this day. However, for higher potencies it is very time consuming, and it is doubtful whether any genuine potencies higher than 1,000c (1M) prepared by the Hahnemann method are available.

In 1832, a Russian general named Korsakov, who was a keen student of homeopathy, recommended a simplified, quicker method. His method employed the *same* glass container, as opposed to Hahnemann's method, which used *different* containers for each serial dilution. He claimed that upon emptying the container after the first dilution, sufficient liquid remained adhering to the walls to be used for the next dilution. For the second centesimal potency, therefore, it was necessary only to add a further 99 parts of alcohol/water to the same container.

Surprisingly, since he usually rejected any deviation from his own procedure, when Korsakov's method was described to Hahnemann, he made the favorable comment that it was "both judicious and useful." It is probable that Hahnemann thought Korsakov's method was irrelevant anyway, as he only prescribed up to 30c potency himself.

The Korsakov method was widely adopted by physicians and pharmacists, and was referred to in many published papers. In 1841, Jahr stated that "for dilutions one does not wish to keep, the obtained dilution can be emptied out and the same flask can be filled with one hundred drops and shaken one hundred times in order to achieve the next dilution. In France, Ecalle-Delpech and Reuvrier described the method in their *Pharmacopoeia*, published in 1854.

Following the teachings of Kent, Swan, Fincke and Skinner in the late 19th century, advocating the use of very high potencies, this increased the use of the Korsakovian method. In some accounts the Hahnemann and Korsakovian methods were mixed, and this led to heated debates among contemporary physicians and pharmacists. Other papers by Kent, Skinner et al., described automatic Korsakovian (continuous fluxion) methods using "dynamizers." Although Berne's work in 1926 proved that the two methods led to considerable difference in concentration, nowadays Hahnemann's method is generally used for preparing potencies up to 200c and the Korsakovian method for higher potencies. Because of the time consuming nature of the Hahnemann method, simple time calculations indicate that it is doubtful whether any potencies higher than 1M claimed to have been produced by the Hahnemann method are geniune. For these potencies, only the Korsakovian method is practical.

Rae Potencies

This method employs a black box device developed Dr. Malcolm Rae in England. Potencies are claimed to be produced by exposing solutions of pure alcohol and water to an electromagnetic field. Its use was banned by the FDA in the United States in 1985. In France the choice does not arise, as French law permits only the Hahnemann method.

NOMENCLATURE OF POTENCIES

A suffix following the potency number indicates the unit steps of dilution and the mode of preparation, thus:

	United States	Great Britain	France
1. Decimal Series	X (or x)	X (or x)	D
2. Centesimal Series			
—Hahnemann	CH (or C or c)	No suffix	CH
—Korsakovian	CK	No suffix	Not
3. Millesimal	m	m	applicable
High Potencies:	1,000 c	1M	
	10,000 c	10M	
	50,000 c	50M	
	100,000 c	CM	

Note: X = Roman numeral for 10
  D = Decimal
  C = Roman numeral for 100
  M = Roman numeral for 1,000

In preparing liquid potencies by either method it is essential that the proper level of alcohol content is maintained. Research at the Royal London Homeopathic Hospital has shown that potencies prepared in water alone lose their therapeutic activity in a few hours.

Succussion

Succussion is the term coined by Hahnemann (probably it was derived from the German *schuffeln* and the Italian *scossone*, meaning to shake violently) for the essential process of violent shaking with impact which follows each step of the sequential dilution, thus completing the potentization procedure. Hahnemann achieved this by holding the vial firmly in his hand and using his forearm to strike a leather bound book. The procedure was repeated at least ten times. Nowadays, mechanical means are usually employed, using instruments of many different designs, all of which aim to simulate the manual procedure. As many as 100 succussions are employed.

One type of mechanical device causes a glass vial, attached to the end of a motor driven rocking arm, to impinge on a rubber pad on each downward stroke.

Not only does succussion ensure an intimate mixing of the

liquid and diluent, but it is also believed it energizes the potency. This potential energy is subsequently released as kinetic energy in the healing process.

Trituration

This process is employed to "solubilize" insoluble minerals and chemical elements in their solid form, that is, to render the crystals or powder to a degree of fineness and subdivision which will permit their solubilization in alcohol/water.

One part (or 1gm) of the substance is finely ground, using a mortar and pestle, with a small part of 99 parts of pure lactose (milk sugar). The trituration is continued for at least one hour, while adding aliquot parts of the remainder of the lactose at 10 to 20 minute intervals. The resultant finely divided powder represents the first centesimal triturated potency. The entire process is repeated, using one part of the first centesimal trituration and a further 99 parts of pure lactose to produce the second centesimal triturated potency, and so on.

For each insoluble mineral or element, a certain potency level is reached, whereby it is sufficiently "diluted" to be within its solubility limit in the alcohol/water. At this stage, higher potencies can be prepared in the liquid form in the usual manner. It follows, therefore, that very low potencies of insoluble substances cannot exist in liquid form. Unscrupulous "manufacturers" of homeopathic medicines have been known to offer customers, for example, *liquid* Graphites 3X!

Potentization Cycle

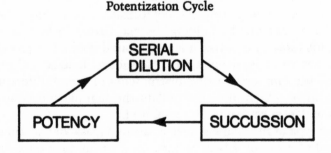

SUMMARY OF POTENCY EQUIVALENTS AND DESIGNATIONS

Hahnemannian Method

Dilution Ratio	Concentration	Decimal Series	Centesimal Series
1:10	10^{-1}	1D or 1X	
1:100	10^{-2}	2D or 2X	1 or 1CH
1:1,000	10^{-3}	3D or 3X	
1:10,000	10^{-4}	4D or 4X	2 or 2CH
1:100,000	10^{-5}	5D or 5X	
1:1,000,000	10^{-6}	6D or 6X	3 or 3CH
1:10^{12}	10^{-12}	12D or 12X	6 or 6CH
1:10^{24}	10^{-24}	24D or 24X	12 or 12CH
1:10^{60}	10^{-60}	60D or 60X	30 or 30CH
1:10^{400}	10^{-400}		200 or 200CH
1:10^{2000}	10^{-2000}		1M or 1,000CH

Avogadro's Hypothesis

In 1811, the Italian physicist Avogadro postulated that equal volumes contain equal numbers of molecules. Therefore, there is a fixed number of molecules (6.4×10^{23}) in unit volume at standard temperature and pressure ($0°$ Celsius, 1.013 N/m^2). Avogadro's hypothesis was proved later by experiment.

It follows, therefore, that the serial or sequential dilution employed in the potentization procedure, ultimately exceeds the Avogadro limit, when *theoretically* none of the original molecules of the original mother tincture remain. In theory, none of the original molecules exist in potencies of 24X or 12CH and higher potencies.

Not surprisingly, this fact was seized upon by the detractors of homeopathy. Trained in the allopathic belief in massive doses of medicine, their credence was already stretched by the infinitely small doses employed in homeopathy, and the suggestion that there may be no actual medicament at all in higher potencies was the last straw.

In 1821, Hahnemann wrote a treatise on the effectiveness of small doses in the 6th volume of his *Materia Medica Pura*. "Some people wonder how it is possible for small doses of extremely rarefied medicines to keep their power (and a great power indeed). This is because they have not understood the word 'Verdünnung' (dilution, rarefaction) which I necessarily had to use when speaking of the preparation of homeopathic medicines. May I answer that the idea is inconceivable only because people have wrong ideas about the essence of medicinal substances."

In his *Treatise of Chronic Diseases*, published in 1832, he was more precise: "The change which is produced by prolonged trituration with a nonmedically active powder or by long shaking-up with an equally nonmedically active liquid is so considerable that it nearly constitutes a miracle. Homeopathy may be proud of having discovered it."

Experiments have shown that, in practice, none of the original molecules of the mother tincture remain even on reaching the 18th potency—well below the theoretical limit of 24X. It is known, however, that there are deviations in the laws of dilution of very high dilutions.

There is, of course, massive clinical evidence of the activity of high potencies and, in certain conditions, an even higher activity than low potencies of the same remedy. In recent years, several research studies have used scientific data in support of the clinical studies, for example, infra-red spectra, intramolecular and intermolecular electronic configurations and nuclear magnetic resonance (See Chapter 5).

The most recent, undisputed clinical evidence was the result of a controlled trial of a 30CH potency of mixed grass pollens in hayfever, published in the *Lancet* (London and Boston) in 1986 (see Chapter 5), which demonstrated its effectiveness compared with placebo unequivocally. The report ended, "The drug we used was potentized to the point where, in theory, none of the original material remained. Yet, these results and those of the pilot study offer no support for the suggestion that the observed effects were wholly due to placebo responses. As such they are a contemporary restatement of an empirical puzzle, now in its second century, and represent a confusing challenge to orthodox scientific models."

QUALITY CONTROL

The manufacture of homeopathic medicines is controlled by the Food and Drug Administration in the United States and Departments of Health in other countries. In Great Britain, manufacture is controlled by the Medicines Act, 1968 and 1971. Nowadays, in the developed countries, all pharmaceutical manufacture is governed by common procedures termed Good Manufacturing Practices (GMP).

These controls ensure stringent standards in relation to buildings, equipment and facilities, qualified staff and quality control procedures. Problems have arisen, in that medicine legislation in most countries was drawn up essentially for allopathic medicines. However, after much discussion, it is now generally agreed that basic scientific techniques and modern laboratory equipment and procedures are equally applicable to homeopathy. Only in a few instances must homeopathic procedures necessarily deviate from the standard approach.

Modern laboratory procedures and systems of quality control do not invalidate Hahnemann's original precepts nor replace classical procedures. Hahnemann wrote: "A dedicated physician can only be sure about the healing properties of a medicine when it is made as pure and as perfect as possible."

Indeed, had modern advances in scientific knowledge and equipment been available to him, he, in his wisdom, would certainly have taken advantage of them. Standards of quality and reproducibility of homeopathic medicines are of fundamental importance to the homeopathic practitioner since he relies on their efficacy. Efficacy and quality of medicines are synonymous.

Quality Control Systems

Rightly, Hahnemann viewed the preparation of the medicines as a science and, as such, it requires a scientific system of quality control.

It must be emphasized however, that ultimately the attainment of a high quality standard is only possible if one can rely on the integrity, the involvement, the training, experience and the commitment of all concerned. This is essentially a team activity in the true spirit of providing a service to homeopathy, and the objective must always be to guarantee the purity, reliability and reproducibility of the medicines supplied to the practitioner.

High standards of personal cleanliness must be maintained by all personnel and hand-washing facilities made available and used regularly.

Protective clothing, including clean overalls and hats, must be worn at all times in manufacturing areas, not only by personnel, but also by visitors entering manufacturing areas. Separate changing rooms are provided for this purpose. Stringent housekeeping methods must be employed and floors regularly washed and all surfaces where dust and dirt may collect wiped regularly. Utensils are washed thoroughly each time after use. Naturally, smoking, drinking and eating are not permitted in manufacturing areas under any circumstances.

The first stage in any quality control system is the transfer of each delivery of incoming raw materials to a Quarantine Store. Each delivery or batch is allocated a reference number which can identify the material through each stage of manufacture. A sample is taken for testing to ensure that it complies with Raw Material Specification in every respect. For example, botanical identification of plant raw materials is carried out and, having established their identity, they are examined for contaminations, such as other plant species, dirt, mold or insects.

Specimens may be dried and pressed for retention or photographed and, in certain circumstances, subjected to microscopic analysis from which microphotographs are taken. Release of all raw materials from the Quarantine Store for use is made only on the authority of the person responsible for quality control and if they are labeled as fit for use. Rejected materials are promptly destroyed. Labels for the finished packed product are also subject to quality control inspection to ensure their accuracy. They are checked for misprints before they are released to the production area.

At the commencement of each manufacturing step, all equipment is inspected to ensure it is clean and free from contamination from any other raw materials or products. At each stage, all materials and equipment are carefully labeled to identify the material being processed and each discrete quantity of raw material or product is labeled with a batch number. Written manufacturing procedures are closely followed in each manufacturing step and batch records are completed, indicating times, temperatures, weights, etc. Thus, the history of each batch, including the utilization of raw materials and even packing materials, may be checked.

At any time during manufacture and packaging of homeopathic medicines, quality control personnel are required to make spot checks and take samples for laboratory analysis, thus monitoring every operation. Particular care is taken in the preparation of mother tinctures and potencies to ensure absolute purity and reproducibility.

On completion of manufacture, representative samples of the finished product are taken according to prescribed procedures and labeled with the batch number and identity. Analytical tests are carried out in the laboratory to ensure that the product meets the Finished Product Specification and then—and only then—is the product finally released from quarantine to the store to await dispatch. Samples of each batch of finished product are always retained in the laboratory. Storage conditions are carefully controlled to ensure that the products do not deteriorate before being passed to the practitioner. Finally, all manufacturing records are checked and filed and all equipment utilized in the manufacture is cleaned in accordance with Cleaning Schedules, which lay down cleaning and inspection operations for each item of equipment.

General precautions to ensure quality, which apply to all manufacturing operations, include the segregation of processing areas to avoid possible cross-contamination, the use of laminar air flow equipment or air conditioning, and all operations carried out in such a way that the risk of contamination is minimized. A recent innovation is microbiological testing by swab or settle plate method to monitor environmental contamination of all manufacturing areas.

Quality Control of Mother Tinctures and Potencies

Concerning homeopathic potencies, this is an area which presents the greatest challenge to the quality analyst. We do not know or understand, yet alone measure, the intrinsic forces or vibrations which may play a part in the healing process of homeopathic potencies. Furthermore, the extremely high dilution of homeopathic potencies makes it almost impossible to apply analytical tests by conventional methods in the laboratory. Even a relatively low potency such as 6x, with concentrations of individual "active ingredients" less than one part per million, is outside the accuracy of many modern instruments. For this reason, only mother tinctures and low potencies (1x, 2x) are subjected to a more comprehensive analysis, both qualitative and quantitative.

Additionally, we have the problem of the chemical complexity of the natural extract contained in the original mother tincture. These may be inorganic or organic, with complex mixtures including minerals, amino acids, proteins, steroids, vitamins, organo-metallic compounds, alkaloids, flavenoids, etc.

This raises a most important point. The conventional allopathic approach to quality control in manufacture is to place great reliance on the assay of the final product, which usually incorporates one or two readily identifiable "active ingredients," all of them at relatively high levels of concentration. Because of the complexity and the high dilution of homeopathic remedies, as described, this approach is not possible and therefore it is considered that "in process" quality control, embracing every step of the preparation from raw material to finished homeopathic medicines is critical in ensuring their purity and safety. It is arguable, therefore, that a system of quality control is even more important than for their allopathic counterparts (see chart on page 63). Ethyl alcohol (94.9 percent by volume), which conforms with the U.S.P. (or B.P.) specifications, must be used in all homeopathic preparations, or preferably distilled grain alcohol. Water must be redistilled using glass or stainless steel equipment with a packed, fractionating column and a reflux ratio of not less than 1:1.

Chemical and Physical Tests

Physical Properties

Mother tinctures and liquid potencies may be tested routinely for their physical properties, including specific gravity, refractive index, and organoleptic tests, such as color and smell.

General Tests

These may include dry residue (total solids), pH, water content by Karl Fischer technique and percentage alcohol content.

Analysis of Chemical Elements

These assays are carried out by conventional chemical methods and can provide a means of identification and a guide to the purity of mother tinctures, and even for low potencies. An example analysis is given below, which illustrates the wide variation between different mother tinctures:

	Crataegus φ	Nux. vom. φ
Iron, parts per million	1.9	0.3
Calcium, parts per million	1,500	1.9
Sodium, parts per million	16.0	6.8
Sulfur, percent	0.003	0.005
Nitrogen, percent	0.005	0.005

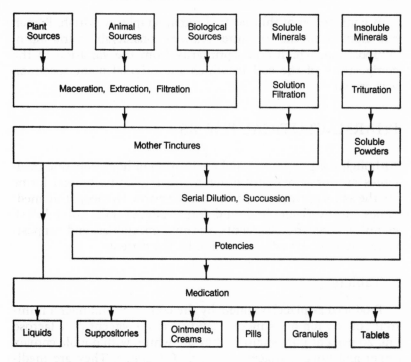

Schematic Diagram of Preparation of Homeopathic Medicines

Other trace elements present in low concentration include zinc, potassium, copper, cobalt, selenium, magnesium and manganese. Differences in assay occur between mother tinctures prepared from plants grown in different locations. For example, a plant grown in limestone soil would be expected to have a higher calcium content than the same species grown in sandy soil.

Thin Layer Chromatography

Thin layer chromotography utilizes the different migration rates of individual constituents of mother tinctures or very low potencies on a thin film of inert material.

This technique is now widely used and shows characteristic bands on a layer of silica gel of 25 to 250 μm thickness, each band representing a specific chemical constituent of the mother tincture. These bands constitute a "thumb print" not only for each mother tincture itself, but also for different batches of the same mother tincture. Various solvent systems have been used, such as butanol/acetic acid or methanol/chloroform over development distances of about 10 cm.

A comparison of thin layer chromatographs of British, French and German mother tinctures showed considerable variation of composition, which arises primarily from the variation in the composition of the soil in which the original plant specimen was grown.

PHARMACEUTICAL FORMS

Although the preparation and application of homoeopathic medicines are fundamentally different, their pharmaceutical forms are the same as their allopathic counterparts. Homeopathic medicines are available in liquid form, tablets, pills (or pilules), granules, powders, ointments, creams, injectables, and suppositories, suitable for administration by the patient.

Tablets

Produced as placebo tablets by the compression under a minimum of one ton pressure of a mixture of 80 percent pure lactose and 20 percent pure sucrose, they are white, with double convex upper and lower surfaces, weighing 0.1 grams. They are medicated by dripping or spraying liquid potencies onto the tablets in such a manner as to ensure a coefficient of impregnation of almost 100 percent. It is essential that liquid potencies used for medication have a high alcohol content (95 percent volume/volume), otherwise they will tend to dissolve the tablet and their stability is impaired.

In certain cases, for example, tissue salts (cell salts, Biochemic remedies, Schuessler salts) triturated powders (usually 6x), are compressed directly.

Pills and Granules

Pills, or pilules, are the traditional homeopathic pharmaceutical form favored by many homeopaths. They are spherical in shape, of about 4 millimeters diameter and 3 to 5 centigrams in weight. In the United States and France, pilules are termed granules.

Granules are also spherical, but smaller than pills, weighing about 5 milligrams. Both placebo pills and granules are prepared from pure lactose by similar procedures. They are medicated in the same manner as tablets.

Ointments, Creams and Suppositories

These pharmaceutical forms, employed only to a limited extent in homeopathy, are prepared in a similar manner to allopathic medicaments. Water-based creams are preferred as they do not stain dressings or clothes.

Ointments and creams are impregnated with a low liquid potency or, sometimes, mother tinctures and are generally prescribed as specific remedies. Examples are Hamamelis Virginiana (alone or in combination with other remedies) for bleeding piles; Arnica for bruises; Calendula Officinalis for minor cuts and sores and Rhus Toxicodendron for rheumatic pain.

Homeopathic suppositories are prepared in the conventional manner. They are impregnated in the same manner as ointments and creams.

Liquids

Liquid potencies are widely used in homeopathy. They are usually supplied in amber glass dropper bottles to protect them from light.

Injectables are also available, but their use is restricted by legislation in many countries.

NOMENCLATURE OF HOMEOPATHIC MEDICINES

Medicines are known internationally by their generic name, in Latin, according to the concise method of naming plant and animal species laid down by the Swedish botanist, Linnaeus (1707–1778).

For example, *Calendula Officinalis*: The first word describes the plant or animal species. The second word describes the particular subspecies of the plant or animal. The common names given to plants are specific to each particular language: in the example given, *Marigold*, in English. Similarly, we have, *Lachesis Muta*, commonly known in English as the Bushmaster Snake (venom).

STABILITY AND STORAGE
OF HOMEOPATHIC MEDICINES

With a relatively low content of medicament, homeopathic medicines are very sensitive. Tablets, pilules or granules must not be touched with the hand as chemicals in the skin such as amino acids, may affect them. The dose should be tipped into the cap of their container and then tipped onto or under the tongue. Alternatively, a clean, dry spoon may be used.

Medicines should be stored in glass containers, in a cool, dry, dark place away from substances with a strong smell, such as garlic or camphor. All containers must be well stoppered.

It is generally accepted for legal purposes that medicines which are properly prepared and stored will have nominal shelf life of about five years. However, the medicines, if properly prepared and stored, *can* retain their activity indefinitely.

Stability and Storage of Mother Tinctures

Some freshly prepared mother tinctures may be supersaturated and, particularly during lengthy storage in a cool place, the clear solution may become cloudy or produce a precipitate which forms a sediment at the bottom of the container. This insoluble matter may simply be filtered off and the clear filtrate will retain the original activity of the mother tincture.

Another cause of a precipitate in a mother tincture may be from the evaporation of alcohol through a badly fitting stopper on the container. In this case, the mother tincture should be rejected.

Mother tinctures must be stored in well-sealed, amber glass bottles in a cool, dark place; they must not be exposed to sunlight. On lengthy storage, tinctures may darken a little without deleterious effect, but if a total color change occurs the material should be rejected, as this is evidence of chemical decomposition of one or more of its constituents.

Quality Criteria of Homeopathic Medicines

Discerning pharmacists and physicians must be aware of the following cautionary points in relation to all homeopathic medicines.

1. Low potency liquids of insoluble substances, such as Graphites 6x, Sulfur 3x or Silica 3x, do not exist and their availability is spurious.

2. High potencies such as 10M, 50M, claimed to have been prepared by Hahnemannian procedures, are of doubtful validity.

3. Certain plastic materials are liable to interact chemically with homeopathic mother tinctures and potencies. This has been demonstrated in experiments using infrared spectroscopic techniques.

4. With the exception of glycerin macerates of gemmotherapy preparations, all homeopathic medicines should have a characteristic alcoholic odor. The presence of alcohol, which is essential for the quality and stability of the medicines, may be determined by organoleptic tests or chemical, physical or electronic tests.

5. Trademarks or proprietary names given to single homeopathic medicines are anathema to homeopathy.

6. Homeopathic medicines, properly prepared and stored, can retain their therapeutic activity indefinitely.

7. All containers of homeopathic medicines must be labeled with the Batch Number or Lot Number, the correct name of the medicines, the potency, the name and address of the manufacturer and a Government Warning, otherwise they are illegal.

SYMBOLS AND ABBREVIATIONS IN HOMEOPATHIC PHARMACY

φ Mother Tincture
MT Mother Tincture
C(or c) Centesimal Potency
X (or x) Decimal Potency
H Hahnemannian
K Korsakovian
M 1,000 or Millesimal Potency
N Potency Number
CH Centesimal Potency by Hahnemannian Method
D Decimal Potency (Europe, except United Kingdom)
Hom. Homeopathy or Homeopathic

Specimen Homeopathic prescriptions are given in Chapter 4. Although the preparation of homeopathic medicines is essentially scientific, the skill and dedication of the pharmacist and scientists are required to capture the essence, the subtlety of their natural sources. Thus, the natural curative powers of the medicines are optimized for the benefit of the patient.

4 HOMEOPATHIC PRESCRIBING

The homeopathic physician is faced with a more difficult task than his allopathic counterpart. He or she must not only make a conventional diagnosis of the patient's condition, but must also base his or her choice of a suitable homeopathic remedy on the total symptom picture and the individuality of the patient. It is for this reason that, at least for the initial consultation, one to two hours may be necessary.

The physician must identify the prime symptoms presented by the patient and their modalities, take into account his past medical and environmental history and consider his physical characteristics, personality and temperament. In this way, the patient's individual characteristics can be identified and his whole person understood and treated. A study of the *Homeopathic Materia Medica* is, therefore, essential. A *Materia Medica* could be described as a series of drug pictures. The original *Materia Medica* was written by Hahnemann, entitled the *Materia Medica Pura*. It was based on Hahnemann's provings of 66 remedies and is still fundamentally important in homeopathic practice.

The following is a typical example, taken from a *Materia Medica* (Boericke):

> CUPRUM ACETICUM (Copper Acetate)
>
> Hay fever, with burning excoriation, paroxysmal cough; tough, tenacious mucus, and fear of suffocation. Protracted labor. Chronic psoriasis and lepra.
>
> *Head*—Violent throbbing and lancinating pains in forehead. Left-sided brow ague. Brain seems void. Inclined to gape and cry. Loses consciousness; head reels when in high-ceiled room. Constant protrusion and retraction of the tongue. Neuralgia with heaviness of head, burning, stinging and stitching in temples and forehead.
>
> *Face*—Collapsed, hippocratic. Facial neuralgia in

69

cheek bone, upper jaw and behind right ear. Better by chewing, pressure and external warmth.

Stomach—Violent spasmodic pains in stomach and abdomen. Vomiting. Slimy brown diarrhea. Violent tenesmus. Cholera.

Respiratory—Attacks of angina pectoris coming on when excited. Violent spasmodic cough. Short, difficult respiration. Spasmodic constriction of chest. Dyspnea.

Skin—Leprous-like eruption, without itching, over whole body, in spots of various sizes.

Modalities—Worse; mental emotions, touch. Better; chewing, pressure, night, lying on affected side and warmth.

Relationship—Acts similarly to Cuprum Met. but is more violent in action.

Dose—Third to sixth trituration.

Homeopathic remedies may be classified according to the manner in which they are prescribed. Thus, we have:

1. The Single Remedy
2. Specific Remedies
3. Polycrest (or Polychrest) Remedies
4. Constitutional Remedies
5. Combination Remedies (Polypharmacy)

THE SINGLE REMEDY

The prescription of a single remedy in accordance with the Law of Similars—"Similia Similibus Curentur"—*is the core of homeopathic practice.* Samuel Hahnemann always advocated the use of a single remedy based on well-defined principles, and he would never countenance two or more remedies administered to the patient *at one time.* The single remedy is chosen by reference to the *Materia Medica* and is aimed at the patient as a whole. This is the classical method of practicing homeopathy.

The prescription of only one remedy at a time was given the name *Kentism* after the teachings of Dr. James Tyler Kent. Adherents to Dr. Kent's teachings are termed Unicists. It must be pointed out, however, that it is not inconsistent with Kentism to prescribe other remedies for the patient if they are administered *at different times* in rotation. Indeed, this method was often used by Hahnemann, for example, in the treatment of cholera.

SPECIFIC REMEDIES

Some single remedies are specific, or more accurately, "near specific," for the treatment of certain strongly indicated symptoms. In these cases, the symptoms are predominant and the constitutional element of the remedy is minimal, that is the remedy will be of some benefit to most people regardless of their physical and mental characteristics. Examples of "near specifics" are:

Remedy	Condition in Which Indicated
Arnica Montana	Bruises
Cantharis Vesicatoria	Burns. Cystitis. Urinary Disorders
Cuprum Metallicum	Cramp
Colchicum Autumnale	Gout
Chamomilla	Teething of infants
Hamamelis Virginiana	Varicose Veins
Urtica Urens	Urticaria
Thuja Occidentalis	Warts
Ignatia Amara	Grief. Bereavement.

POLYCREST (OR POLYCHREST) REMEDIES

The polychrests, so named by Hahnemann (from the Greek *polychrestos*—"many uses"), are a range of frequently used remedies prescribed for a wide spectrum of clinical symptoms. In this sense, they are more symptom oriented, although the physical and mental characteristics of the patient still influence the final choice.

Polychrest remedies include many of the classic homeopathic remedies such as Aconite, Arnica, Arsen Alb., Belladonna, Bryonia, Carbo Veg., Causticum, Chamomilla, Gelsemium, Graphites, Ignatia, Lachesis, Lycopodium, Natrium Mur., Phosphorus, Pulsatilla, Sepia, Silica, Sulfur and Thuja.

CONSTITUTIONAL REMEDIES

There are several definitions of a constitutional remedy, which might be described as a remedy prescribed in a person-oriented manner. The concept is that certain people have a special affinity to a particular remedy and respond to it for a variety of conditions. In this case, the person is predominant and the remedy is prescribed on the basis of the type of patient rather than on the clinical symptoms. Thus, the whole personality of the patient is taken into account—his or her temperament, fears, emotions, likes and dislikes, moods and lifestyle. The constitutional remedy aims to capture the whole ethos of the patient.

The constitutional remedy was not part of Hahnemann's basic teaching, but rather a concept introduced in the early 20th century by Dr. Kent in the United States, and followed by other homeopathic physicians, including Dr. Margaret Tyler and Dr. Margery Blackie in England.

Thus, we have constitutional types, such as the *Pulsatilla type* or the *Graphites type*. These individuals are said to have a special affinity to these medicines. Examples are as follows:

Graphites Type   A fat, flabby person with an extremely cautious nature. Has a pale, unhealthy skin, is subject to flatulence and constipation and is susceptible to cold. In the woman, menstruation is late and breasts are large and hard; frigidity is frequent.

Pulsatilla Type   This is a classic case, often quoted. Females, particularly young girls, with blonde or light brown hair, blue eyes and a pale, delicate complexion. She is gentle, fearful, friendly but shy. Romantic and emotional she easily becomes weepy, even on a slight reprimand. She dislikes cold, but seeks cool places. Her problems are not helped by using oral contraceptives.

Sepia Type   The Sepia type of person, of either sex, is thin, dark haired and often below average height. Tends to be indolent and fearful. Sepia women are easily depressed. They have a dislike of fatty and starchy foods and milk.

Nux Vomica Type   The Nux Vomica type is easily recognized. His physical characteristics may be quite different, but he is more likely to be dark haired and thin. He is aggressive, bellicose, ambitious and hyperactive. His depressive moods are worse between 3 a.m. and 4 a.m. He seeks stimulation with alcohol and is subject to hangovers. Nux Vomica is suitable for drug addicts.

Lycopodium Type   May be tall and thin with sallow complexion and freckles. Intellectual people lacking in physical stamina. Conscientious and sensitive, they are subject to worry and fears, particularly over responsibilities, but can be headstrong.

Lachesis Type   Jealousy and suspicion dominate this person. Excitable, talkative person, possibly with freckles and red hair, with tendency to blue or purple coloration of affected skin.

Sulfur Type Lean, dyspeptic, nervous person, often appearing disheveled and inclined to be selfish. Unhealthy, hard looking skin, with tendancy to skin diseases and perspires easily with body odor. Red orifices. Deep thinking people who meditate and philosophize. Likes to be independant.

Ignatia Type The patient is nervous and inclined to be neurotic. He or she is emotional and sensitive; mental state alters rapidly. A dislike of tobacco smoke is not uncommon and patient is often tearful.

Leuticum Type This person may have a family history of syphilis. Thin and weak, fearful and has a bad memory.

COMBINATION REMEDIES

A combination, or mixture, of several different remedies administered to the patient at the same time, known as polypharmacy. Combinations of as many as ten remedies may be employed, but generally they number between five and seven remedies, often in different but low potencies. Their choice is designed to match the totality of symptoms of an illness.

The totality of symptoms of a disease (S_t) may be represented mathematically as follows:

$$S_t = (S_1, S_2, S_3, \ldots\ldots\ldots\ldots\ldots S_n)$$

The symptoms S_1, S_2, etc. include the physical, mental, general and particular symptoms of the patient.

Combinations are strongly criticized by strict homeopaths, who point out that this practice is contrary to Hahnemann principles. It is said by some that the combination remedy is the "blunderbuss" approach, compared with the accurate "rifle" of the single remedy. It is fair to record, however, that many homeopathic practitioners favor the combination remedy and provide ample demonstrations of their effectiveness.

The actual remedies selected for a combination remedy require considerable skill in achieving a synergistic effect. We know that certain remedies antidote other remedies, and in effect cancel one another out. Some remedies complement one anther, by reinforcing the activity of another remedy. Practitioners who prescribe combination remedies are known as "Complexists."

Examples of the relationship of some commonly used medicines are given below:

Remedy	Complementary Remedies	Antidotes	
Aconite	Arnica	Belladonna	
		Berberis	
	Sulfur	Nux Vomica	
Arnica	Aconite	Arsen Alb.	
	Ipecacuanha	Camphor	
	Hypericum	Ignatia	
	Rhus Tox.		
Belladonna	Calc. Carb.	Aconite	
	Calc. Fluor.	Merc. Sol.	
	Calc. Phos.	Hepar Sulf.	
Bryonia	Rhus Tox.	Aconite	Nux Vomica
	Alum	Camphor	Pulsatilla
		Chamomilla	Ignatia
		Chelidonium	
Calc. Carb.	Belladonna	Bryonia	Nux Vomica
	Rhus Tox.	Camphor	Sepia
		Ipecacuanha	Sulfur
Graphites	Arsen Alb.	Aconite	
	Causticum	Nux Vomica	
	Hepar Sulf.		
	Lycopodium		
Lachesis	Hepar Sulf.	Alum	Carbo Veg.
	Lycopodium	Belladonna	Nux Vomica
		Cocculus	
Ruta Grav.	Calc. Phos.	Camphor	
Sepia	Nux Vomica	Aconite	
	Natrium Mur.	Sulfur	
	Sabadilla	Antim. Crud.	
Sulfur	Aconite	Aconite	Pulsatilla
	Nux Vomica	Chamomilla	Rhus Tox.
	Psorinum	Causticum	Sepia
		Nux Vomica	Silica
		Merc. Sol.	

Antidotes are sometimes prescribed to eliminate the excessive aggravation of another remedy.

Typical combination remedies and their indications are as follows:

Travel Sickness and Nausea (Dolisos)
Belladonna 6x
Colchicum Autumnale 6x
Cocculus Indicus 6x
Ipecacuanha 6x
Nux Vomica 6x
Petroleum 6x
Tabacum 6x

Hay Fever-Like Symptoms (Dolisos)
Allium Cepa 3x
Ambrosia 3x
Apis Mellifica 6x
Euphrasia 3x
Formica Rufa 6x
Sabadilla 3x

Cough and Sore Throat (Longevity)
Spongia Tosta 3x
Phosphorus 6x
Coccus Cacti 6x
Ipecacuanha 6x
Hepar Sulfuris Calcareum 6x
Drosera Rotundifola 6x
Belladonna 12x
Aconitum Napellus 12x

Headache (Longevity)
Bryonia Alba 6x
Cimifuga Racemosa 6x
Glonoinum 6x
Iris Versicolor 6x
Sanguinaria Canadensis 6x
Apis Mellifica 6x
Belladonna 12x

A variation of the combination remedy principle is the administration of two or more different potencies of the same remedy at the same time. For example, Arnica 6x and Arnica 30x.

NOSODES AND ISODES

Nosodes

Nosodes were originally introduced by Dr. Edward Bach in England and Dr. John Paterson in Glasgow, Scotland.

Nosodes are remedies derived from diseased tissues, for example pus, which are potentized in the normal way and, therefore, contain no active organisms. They are used primarily in prophylaxis and as an initial remedy when the symptom picture is unclear, but are finding increasing use as a follow-up treatment to acute infectious illness. Their prophylactic use is the homeopathic equivalent to vaccination.

Nosodes are usually prescribed in a single dose at the 30th centesimal potency, but never less than the 12th centesimal potency. They are often prescribed when the patient complains of "never being well since. . . ."

Certain nosodes have a complete drug picture and these are based on provings, and featured fully in the *Materia Medica*. They may, therefore, be selected in the conventional manner. Examples are:

Medorrhinum (gonorrhea)
Tuberculinum (tuberculosis)
Syphilinum (syphilitic virus)
Psorinum (scabies vesicle)

Other nosodes have a limited symptom picture and limited provings. Examples are:

Influenzinum (influenza)
Diptherinum (diptheritic virus)
Anthracinum (anthrax)
Parotidinum (mumps)

Influenzinum is often prescribed in the form of a mixture of several common strains of influenza virus, as a prophylactic.

Bowel Nosodes are remedies derived from cultures of stools containing intestinal bacteria.

They are usually prescribed in a single dose at the 30th centesimal potency, although a second dose is sometimes given after several months, other conventional remedies being given in the meantime. Nowadays they are chosen on the basis of specific clinical indications or being complementary to other remedies. Examples of bowel nosodes are:

Morgan Co. (Bach) (Morgan Pure or Morgan Gaertner)
Proteus
Sycotic Co.
Bacillus No. 7

The suffix *inum* is used in the nomenclature of most nosodes, but is not exclusive to nosodes.

A full list of nosodes and bowel nosodes is given in Appendix 1.

From his extensive clinical and laboratory observations over 20 years (not Hahnemann's provings), Dr. Paterson demonstrated that the non-lactose fermenting bacilli of the bowel is biochemically related to the disease and the homeopathic remedy. Each germ was associated with its own peculiar symptom picture or disease. He concluded that: 1) the specific organism is related to the disease; 2) the specific organism is related to the homeopathic remedy; 3) the homeopathic remedy is related to the disease.

The potentized nosode prepared from the culture of the organism can be considered to be a complex biochemical substance having the characteristic of the disturbed metabolism, and thus to be similar to the disease, and, according to the

Law of Similars, to have specific therapeutic power to restore balance.

Paterson recorded that the bowel nosodes are deep and broad-acting remedies covering the totality of symptoms from the highest mental levels to the lowest "gross pathology" level and, in taking the case history, attention must be given to the past as well as the present symptoms.

Where a definite symptom picture points to a particular remedy, then this remedy should be prescribed. If the choice lies with a number of remedies, then these remedies may be used with the associated bowel nosodes. For example, if Calcarea Carbonica, Sulfur and Graphites were the possible remedies, Morgan Pure (Paterson) is related to each of these remedies and could cover the totality of the symptoms.

The number and frequency of the doses of bowel nosodes may be determined by clinical experience, but the dose should not be repeated within three months. Bowel nosodes, if properly used, are considered to be valuable remedies, particularly in the treatment of chronic disease and in cases resistant to any other form of treatment.

Isodes

Isotherapy, or *Isopathy*, is the practice of treating diseases with homeopathic potencies derived from the causative agent of the disease *taken from the patient*. They bear a relationship, therefore, to the nosodes.

Isotherapeutic agents are called *isodes*. Isodes are often employed in the treatment of allergies. Thus, we may treat hay fever sufferers with potencies of certain types of grass, pollen or house dust. A double-blind, controlled clinical trial carried out by D. Reilly, M. Taylor, et al. in 1986 showed that a potency of mixed grass pollens significantly reduced hay fever symptoms compared with placebo. By this concept, any allergic condition which is associated with a particular substance may be treated with minute homeopathic doses of that substance (the allergen).

Allergens are usually prescribed in 24x, 30CH potency or higher.

A list of typical allergens is given in Appendix 2.

Sarcodes are homeopathic preparations of healthy organs, glands or tissues removed from cattle, sheep or pigs. See Organotherapy, Chapter 5.

MODALITIES

We have seen that modalities are influences that qualify the significant symptoms experienced by the patient, either by worsening them or improving them. Modalities are, therefore, modifying influences which assist the individualized treatment of the patient. A modality can decide between two or more remedies which are strongly indicated on other grounds.

Worsening of symptoms is known as an *aggravation*, which is denoted by the sign <.

Improvement of symptoms is known as *amelioration*, which is denoted by the sign >.

Modalities may be classified as follows:

1. *Physical Modalities:* Touch; rest; exertion; exercise; position of body; movement.
2. *Temperature Modalities:* Cold; warmth; climate.
3. *Time Modalities:* Season of year; day; night; afternoon; evening; hour.
4. *Dietary Modalities:* Food; drink; alcohol.
5. *Localized Modalities or Lateralities:* Right-sided; left-sided; right side to left side; left side to right side; spread in all directions.
6. *Miscellaneous Modalities.*

The modalities of specific homeopathic remedies are as follows:

1. Physical Modalities

Many remedies exhibit physical modalities. The major remedies are listed below:

a) Touch

Better for:	Worse for:	
Bryonia	Arnica	Phosphorus
Colocynth	Apis Mel.	Zincum Met.
Calc. Carb.	Cantharis	Croton Tig.
China	Ferrum Phos.	Belladonna
Chelidonium	Hepar Sulf.	Bryonia
	Lachesis	Spigelia
	Hypericum	Cocculus

b) Movement

Better for:	Worse for:
Bromum	Arnica
Ferrum Phos.	Baptisia

Dulcamara	Bryonia
Lycopodium	Phytolacca
Acidum Nit.	Spigelia
Rhus Tox.	Veratrum Alb.
Pulsatilla	Belladonna
Calc. Fluor.	Nux Vomica
Aurum Met.	Causticum
Pyrogenium	Sabina
Natrum Carb.	Viscum Alb.

c) Rest

Better for:	*Worse for:*
Bryonia	Rhus Tox.
Belladonna	Pulsatilla
Nux Vomica	Lycopodium
Antim. Crud.	Calc. Fluor.
Kali Phos.	

d) Sitting

Better for:	*Worse for:*
Bryonia	Pulsatilla
Nux Vomica	Rhus Tox.
Kali Carb.	Sepia
	Natrum Carb.

e) Lying Down

	Better for:	*Worse for:*	
On either side	Bryonia	Arsen Alb.	Belladonna
	Nux Vomica	Chamomilla	Natrum Mur.
	Arnica	Lycopodium	Mang. Acet.
		Rhus Tox.	Hyoscymus
On left side		Bromum	
		Viscum Alb.	
On right side:	Sulfur	Argentum Nit.	
	Spigelia	Mercurius Sol.	
	Natrum Mur.	Sanguinaria	
On affected side	Bryonia	Aconite	
	Calc. Carb.	Phosphorus	
	Ignatia	Hepar Sulf.	
	Pulsatilla	Baryta Carb.	

f) Exercise or Exertion

	Better for:	*Worse for:*	
	Bromum	Bryonia	Cad. Sulf.
	Juglans Cin.	Kali Phos.	Phos. Acidum
	Mag. Carb.	Calc. Carb.	Phosphorus
	Rhus Tox.	Calc. Ars.	
	Fluor. Acidum		

g) *Ascending Stairs*

Worse for:
Phosphorus
Spongia

h) *Bending Forward*

Better for: Worse for:
Kali Carbonica   Hypericum
Colocynthis
Hyoscyamus

2. Temperature Modalities

These modalities are probably the most important consideration in the choice of the correct remedy.

a) *Warmth*

Better for: Worse for:
Arsenicum Alb.   Chamomilla
Belladonna   Apis Mel.
Calc. Carb.   Ledum
Aurum Met.   Pulsatilla
Causticum   Sulfur
Drosera   Secale
Kali Bich.   Allium Cepa
Nux Vomica   Fluoricum Acidum
Kali Phos.   Aconite
Lycopodium   Antimonium Crudum
Rhus Tox.   Chamomilla
Sepia   Bryonia
Silica
Veratrum Alb.

b) *Cold*

Better for: Worse for:
Baptisia   Arsen Alb.   Nux Vomica
Bryonia   Calc. Carb.   Lycopodium
Antimonium Tart.   Calc. Fluor.   Sepia
Carbo Veg.   Calc. Phos.   Silica
Lachesis   Causticum   Rhus Tox.
Gelsemium   Arnica   Hypericum
Natrum Mur.   Hepar Sulf.   Ruta Grav.
Pulsatilla   Graphites   Spongia
Allium Cepa   Dulcamara   Aconite
Aloe
Apis Mel.

c) Climate

	Better for:	Worse for:	
Damp weather	Alumina	Natrum Sulf.	Bromum
		Dulcamara	Carbo Veg.
		Rhus Tox.	Calc. Carb.
		Thuja	Calc. Fluor.
Dry weather	Calc. Carb.	Causticum	
		Hepar Sulf.	
		Nux Vomica	
Wind		Nux Vomica	
		Lycopodium	
		Phosphorus	
Cold wind		Bellis	
		Hepar Sulf.	
Storm		Phosphorus	
Warm weather		Borax	

3. Time Modalities

Timetable for symptoms at the peak of their activity.

a) Day/Night/Evening

Worse during night	Worse during day	Worse during evening
Arsen Alb.	Sulfur	Euphrasia
Chamomilla	Natrum Mur.	Phosphorus
Aurum Met.		
Graphites		
Hepar Sulf.		
Rhus Tox.		
Pulsatilla		
Kali Carb.		
Lachesis		
Psorinum		
Calc Carb.		
Aconite		
Dulcamara		
Veratrum Alb.		
Hyoscyamus		

b) Morning/Afternoon

Worse during morning	Worse during afternoon
Sepia	Lycopodium
Lachesis	Belladonna
Natrum Mur.	Causticum
Nux Vomica	Phosphorus

Ignatia   Pulsatilla
Alumina   Cocculus
Fluoricum Acidum
Carbo Veg.
Kali Phos.

c) Hourly

N. B. All times are approximate.

Worse at:

Midnight	Rhus Tox.
Midnight to	
3 a.m.	Drosera
1 to 2 a.m.	Arsen Alb.
Before 3 a.m.	Nux Vomica
	Thuja
2 to 3 a.m.	Kali Bich.
3 a.m.	Bryonia
	Thuja
3 to 4 a.m.	Hypericum
	Ammonium Carb.
4 to 6 a.m.	Ferrum Phos.
9 a.m.	Chamomilla
10 to 11 a.m.	Gelsemium
	Natrum Mur.
11 a.m.	Ipecac.
	Sulfur
2 p.m.	Calc. Carb.
3 p.m.	Belladonna
	Thuja
4 p.m.	Pulsatilla
4 to 5 p.m.	Carbo Veg.
4 to 6 p.m.	Apis Mel.
4 to 8 p.m.	Lycopodium
5 to 6 p.m.	Hepar Sulf.
7 p.m.	Rhus Tox.
9 p.m.	Bryonia
10 p.m. to	
midnight	Belladonna
Before midnight	Aconite
	Graphites
	Pulsatilla

d) Season

Worse during:

Spring	Lachesis
Summer	Gelsemium
	Croton Tig.
Fall	Rhus Tox.
	Thuja
	Merc. Viv.

Winter	Hepar Sulf.	Aurum Met.
	Silica	Viscum Alb.

4. Dietary Modalities

All modalities of food or drink are aggravations. Worse for:

a) Food

Fatty foods	Carbo Veg.	
	Thuja	
Cold foods	Arsen Alb.	Rhus Tox.
	Lycopodium	Pulsatilla
	Nux Vomica	Phosphorus
Sweet foods, sugar	Argent. Nit.	
	Sanguinaria	
Butter	Carbo Veg.	
Pork	Carbo Veg.	
	Pulsatilla	
Fruits	Bryonia	
	Cinchona	
Bread	Bryonia	
	Pulsatilla	

b) Drink

Milk	Carbo Veg.	
Coffee	Nux Vomica	Ignatia
	Causticum	Carbo Veg.
	Chamomilla	Thuja
Beer	Nux Vomica	
	Kali Bich.	
Alcohol	Nux Vomica	Arnica
	Lachesis	Carbo Veg.
	Silica	Arsen Alb.
	Zincum Met.	Antim. Crudum

5. Localized Modalities (Lateralities)

Certain remedies predominantly affect one side of the body, either the left side or the right side of the patient. Thus, we regard them as *right-sided remedies* or *left-sided remedies*. Some symptoms may start at the right side and spread to the left and vice versa; other symptoms shift from side to side of the body.

Left side	Natrum mur.
	Bellis
	Lachesis

	Argentum Nit.
	Berberis
	Surfur
	Dulcamara
Right side	Arsen Alb.
	Kali Carb.
	Lycopodium
	Apis Mel.
Right to left side	Lycopodium
Left to right side	Lachesis
In all directions	Dioscorea

6. Miscellaneous Modalities

There are some modalities which cannot be classified, but their specificity may provide an important pointer to the selection of a remedy. Examples are:

Worse for sexual excesses	Phosphoricum Acidum
Worse for sight or sound of	
running water	Hydrophobinum
Worse for music	Natrum Carb., Aconite
Worse for noise	Natrum Mur.
Better in dark	Phosphorus

Case Histories

Dr. J. H. Clark, in *The Prescriber*, quoted a classic case demonstrating the value of modalities. A 60-year-old female had been troubled with pain for almost 25 years, affecting the right side of her head and right cheek. There were violent pains, shooting in the temple and sudden pains in the cheek, burning like fire. It was worse while eating, worse from touch and better after eating. It was worse when the patient was chilled and sometimes worse at night.

The condition was diagnosed as neuralgia. Consideration of the localized modality, the suddenness, the aggravation by eating and the least movement and touch and at night, Lycopodium Clavatum 200CH was prescribed and the patient's pain was relieved "in a most wonderful way."

A female patient, aged 44, suffered from migraine when under stress over a period of five years and the attacks were more frequent in the last six months. She had no apparent allergies and there was no family history of migraine. She was a shy, emotional person. Menstruation was regular and normal. She disliked heat and felt better in cold. Pulsatilla 30CH with Bryonia 30CH at the onset of a migraine was prescribed. The intensity and frequency of the migraines decreased and cleared altogether after six months.

John, aged 18, suffered from eczema, with itchy eruptions on both hands, for four years. He was a friendly, gregarious person but his dress was untidy. He perspired easily and the palms of his hands were moist. Sulfur 30CH was prescribed and the condition cleared within six weeks.

Maria, aged 35, complained of severe pains in the joints, especially the toes and ankles. She had been on cortisone therapy for eight weeks, with little effect. She was of a nervous disposition, anxious and sometimes irritable or depressed. She was a chilly person with a good appetite, but craved warm drinks and candies. The pain was worse with touch or motion and she felt better in warmth. Carboneum Sulph. 6CH was prescribed with consideration of matching symptoms and modalities in the *Materia Medica* and constitutional factors. After six weeks, the pain was reduced, the patient was no longer depressed and cortisone was reduced to one-third of the original dose. After a further eight weeks, there was no pain in the joints and the cortisone was stopped altogether. The patient was quite mobile with little anxiety.

A male patient, aged 51, was admitted to hospital with a fractured sternum and ribs after a traumatic car accident. The impact of the collision had caused him to bite deep into his tongue. Ater two days of allopathic treatment, his tongue was still painful, swollen and with suppuration. Homeopathic treatment was given on the third day with tincture of Calendula and Hypericum, diluted in three parts of water three times each day. Within two days the tongue was no longer swollen, there was no pus, it gave no pain and healing was well advanced.

A young child, James, was suffering from headaches, as a dull ache particularly on the right side of the forehead. He was thin, with a pale complexion, lacking in confidence, diffident and worried over his schoolwork. He craved sweet foods and hot drinks, but was liable to digestive upsets, particularly late afternoons or early evening. He preferred the open air and disliked hot, stuffy rooms. Lycopodium 30CH was prescribed. The frequency and intensity of his headaches were reduced immediately and stopped altogether after a few days.

POTENCY

Having selected the correct remedy according to the principle of the Similumum and taking into account the individuality of the patient, the appropriate potency is chosen.

It must be stated at this juncture that, in spite of the importance of potency, the selection of the correct remedy is paramount. Thus, the administration of the correct remedy will always be of some benefit to the patient, regardless of potency. It follows that the wrong remedy will be of no benefit. Selection of the appropriate potency will optimize the curative effect of the right remedy.

Common Potencies

The most commonly prescribed potencies are as follows:

Low Potencies: 3x *6x 12x 6CH* 24x 30x
Intermediate Potencies: *30CH (200CH)*
High Potencies: *200CH* 1M 10M 50M CM

Potencies in italic type are most used. Details of dilutions of these potencies are given in Chapter 3. For the reasons explained, it is not valid to interchange potencies of, say, 60x and 30CH, although their dilutions are the same.

Biotherapeutic preparations (see Chapter 5) are prescribed in specific potencies thus:

Gemmotherapeutic preparations are prescribed only in 2x (or 2D) potency.

Organotherapeutic preparations are prescribed in potencies of 4CH, 5CH, 7CH, 9CH, or 30CH.

Lithotherapeutic preparations are prescribed only in 8x potency.

Cook's Hypothesis

Most homeopathic physicians accept that the most commonly prescribed potencies generally correspond to the levels of optimum therapeutic effectiveness for most homeopathic medicines. Research has supported this view; for example the work of Jones and Jenkins (1983) with wheat and yeast growth (see Chapter 5).

The author has put forward (1982) a hypothesis which may explain Hahnemann's original choice of these potencies. It is significant that these chosen potencies were 3, 6, 12, 24 and

30—*all subunits or multiples of the numbers 6 and 12.* Numerical systems based on multiples of 6 or 12 were very common in Europe in Hahnemann's time. The old system, based on units of twelve, is known as the duodecimal system. Hahnemann's own Saxon coinage was based on a major gold coin worth twelve lesser coins.

Similarly, the British coinage, even as late as 1969, was based on 12 pence equal to one shilling (5p). Again, we have 12 inches to one foot. Even the game of tennis, originating in medieval France, has a winning score of 60 (5 x 12) points. It is reasonable to suppose, therefore, that the numbers 3, 6, 12, 24, 30, etc., in everyday use at that time, influenced Hahnemann's choice of logical potency steps. Extrapolating this arithmetical progression suggests that a study of the efficacy of potencies, such as 24, 36, 42, 48, may be useful.

If the foregoing is a valid argument, then why are the most commonly prescribed *higher* potencies, that is 200, 1,000(1M), 10,000(10M) etc, based on the metric system, in units and subunits of 10?

The author has suggested the explanation that higher potencies came into use following the teachings of Drs. Kent, Swan, et. al. in the United States, in the late 19th and early 20th centuries. By this time, the metric system of units had been generally adopted in favor of the old duodecimal system, both in the fields of medicine and science. It is logical, therefore, that Hahnemann's successors would specify *metric* numbers when introducing higher potencies into homeopathic practice.

Another question now arises. Having used the numerical system on multiples of 6 in *prescribing* potencies, why did Hahnemann then use the metric system for the *preparation* of potencies, namely the decimal and centesimal series of dilutions?

The answer may be that Hahnemann was known to regard the *practice* of homeopathy as an *art*. For example, his quintessential work is entitled *The Organon of the Healing Art*. On the other hand, he recognized the preparation of the remedies as an exact *science*. It is reasonable to suppose, therefore, that he chose the scientific metric system, which was already in use in his favorite science—chemistry—for the *preparation* of homeopathic potencies.

Selecting the Potency

There is a wide diversity of opinion among homeopathic practitioners as to the correct potency to employ for a specific case. Those who rely on high potencies would agree that very low potencies are close to allopathic doses, indicating a lack of conviction in homeopathy on the part of the practitioner. Those who rely on low potencies would argue that very high potencies—far beyond the existence of a material dose—are stretching credulity in homeopathy.

Generally, low potencies are most useful in acute conditions and are taken frequently over a short period until the condition improves. For acute conditions, dosing may be given every 2 or 4 hours for up to 12 hours, then 3 times a day between meals. High potencies are most often prescribed for chronic conditions and taken at longer intervals of 3 times a day, once a day, or on a constitutional basis, even once a week. These directions were set out by Hahnemann in the *Organon*.

In some cases, it may be efficacious to start with a lower potency and progressively increase the potency if no improvement is noted.

A view commonly held is that low potencies (6x, 12x, 6CH) are aimed at treating the patient at the physical level, while high potencies (200CH, 1M) are aimed at the mental level and very high potencies (50M, CM), the spiritual level.

Dosing Frequency

General rules which affect the frequency of dosing are as follows:

1. Frequency of dosing is determined, *inter alia*, by the reaction time. For example, Aconite, which is of brief reaction time, may be given more frequently than say, Graphites, which has a longer duration.

2. When improvement is noted, the interval between doses is increased.

3. When the condition is cleared or greatly improved, dosing is stopped.

4. If an aggravation occurs, this, of course, may be a positive sign, but the dosing must be stopped until it has subsided.

5. In the event of another condition arising during treatment, a different remedy should be given.

Note: In certain cases it may be advantageous to alternate remedies, but, in general, a single strongly indicated remedy is preferable.

Dosage

The recommended dose for any remedy in granule (pill or pilule in the United Kingdom) form is 4 granules dissolved slowly under the tongue. The dose for children is 2 granules. The recommended dose for any remedy in tablet form is 2 tablets for adults, 1 tablet for children, dissolved slowly under the tongue.

The recommended dose for remedies in liquid form is 10 drops under the tongue, and for children, 5 drops.

Remedies are best taken between meals, when the mouth and tongue are clean and free from tobacco or highly flavored toothpaste.

DIET AND EXERCISE

Drawing on his experience as Medical Officer of Health for the city of Dresden, Samuel Hahnemann wrote in his book, *The Friend of Health*, published in 1795, of the desirability of plenty of fresh air, a sensible diet, exercise and free movement and adequate rest. This advice was to be a recurring theme in his subsequent essays and, as in most of his medical teachings, he was far ahead of his time. While he was in practice in his last years in Paris, he invariably gave his patients a diet sheet along with the medicine. Proper diet, exercise and sleep must be concomitant with a course of homeopathic medicine to bring the body and mind into harmony with nature and thus optimize the efficacy of the treatment.

ELECTRODIAGNOSIS

Based on a theoretical model from Japanese scientists and a practical application by the German physician Dr. Rheinhold Voll, electrodiagnosis provides a means for evaluating the electromagnetic system of the body.

Impedance to the balanced electrical circulation of the body results in clinical pathology and illness, regardless of the origin. Acupuncture "points" are light emitting diodes (LED) and are specific areas of communication with the surrounding environment. The body resists intrusion from external electrical sources. When approximately 0.9 volts of direct current is introduced into the body surface probe (noninvasive) at specific acupuncture points, the ability of the body to react (resist) in a healthy manner can be determined. Measuring the body's response at specific acupuncture points provides a means of localizing interference fields (patterns) at specific sites of the body (organs, tissues, systems, etc.) for accurate diagnosis.

The introduction of electromagnetic patterns of various homeopathic remedies (including nosodes, isodes and sarcodes) into the terrain of the patient provides the physician with a means for the selection of one or more remedies. These remedies are found to eliminate the current impedance or lack of resistance, both reflecting abnormal body conditions.

The exact potency of each remedy can be determined and prescribed with the prevention of unpleasant aggravations. Also, the compatibility of remedies can be assessed by testing pairs or groups of remedies together at specific acupuncture points.

Electrodiagnosis provides the physician with a unique method of measuring the finite electromagnetic influences continually in operation throughout the body. Such a system offers greater accuracy and a more rapid diagnostic capability.

Current techniques in electrodiagnosis owe much to the work of Dr. Fuller Royal and his associates at the Nevada Clinic of Preventive Medicine in Las Vegas, Nevada.

SPECIMEN HOMEOPATHIC PRESCRIPTIONS

Although standard dosages are given below, it must be remembered that homeopathic medicines act qualitatively rather than quantitatively. Even though the dosage may be exceeded, the medicines are safe from unwanted side effects.

Generally, the dose for children is one half of the adult dose.

1. Granules (Pills or Pilules)

May be supplied in glass or plastic tubes containing approximately 80 granules or 1 oz. bottles containing approximately 250 granules.

Dose: Five granules placed under the tongue and allowed to dissolve slowly. Not to be swallowed or the effectiveness will be reduced. Do not handle the granules—dispense from the lid of the container or from a clean, dry spoon.

Example A: Arnica 6CH, 1 oz. gran. (or 250 granules) 5 every 15 min. for 4 doses, then 2 hourly for 4 doses.

Example B: Belladonna 30CH, 80 granules, 5 every 4 hours then t.d.s. (three times a day) for 3 days.

2. Tablets

Like granules, the tablet form may be prescribed if needed over a long period or for acute conditions.

Tablets may be crushed on a clean spoon for infants. Allow tablets to dissolve slowly under the tongue. Do not handle the tablets—dispense from the lid of the container or from a clean, dry spoon. Do not use if discolored.

Example A: Ruta Grav 6CH, 1 oz. tabs.; 2 to be taken after meals.

Example B: Calc. Carb. 6x, 1 oz. tabs.; 2 to be taken t.d.s. (three times a day) after meals.

3. Liquids and Mother Tinctures

Usually supplied in 1 oz. (30ml) or 2 oz. (60ml) amber glass dropper bottles.

Liquids are dropped directly on or under the tongue, using the glass dropper.

Example A: Crataegus ø—2 drops, ex aq., n. & m. (night and morning).

Example B. Gelsemium 12x—10 drops, ex aq., b.i.d. (twice a day).

4. Ointments

Usually prepared with mother tincture or low potencies (less than 6x).

Example: Arnica ung. (ointment) m.d.u. (to be used as directed.)

When the patient's condition improves, the interval between doses is increased and the treatment is stopped after about two more days.

If aggravation of the symptoms is noticeable the dosing must be stopped until the aggravation has passed.

Treatment is stopped when the condition has completely cleared and restarted only if original symptoms recur. Proper diet and adequate exercise and rest during treatment are strongly recommended.

On setting up homeopathic practice, it is advisable to select, say, 20 or 30 remedies, possibly polychrests, and aim to become thoroughly conversant with them. The practitioner is then able to expand his or her repertory as his or her knowledge and confidence grow.

Constant reference to the *Homeopathic Materia Medica* is necessary to achieve a thorough understanding of each remedy. In treating the whole person it is necessary to know the "whole remedy" with all its nuances and subtlety.

In the foregoing chapters, the author has tried not to be dogmatic, or favor any particular facet of homeopathic practice. Each has its own merits and demerits, and it is for the reader to decide on his or her own particular approach. Homeopathy is a dynamic and flexible therapy and to adopt a narrow, doctrinaire view is to deny its true potential.

The practice of homeopathy is not a sterile, mechanical exercise; it calls for total involvement. Homeopathy is a fascinating, exacting discipline demanding total application, but the intangible rewards are limitless.

5 RESEARCH AND DEVELOPMENT

The basic principle of homeopathy enunciated by Samuel Hahnemann—*Similia Similibus Curentur*, or the *Law of Similars*—is clearly understood and valid both scientifically and medically. Modern homeopathic research is, therefore, broadly centered on three areas:

1. Extension of the Homeopathic Materia Medica by Proving New Drugs

By definition, any substance capable of inducing disease symptoms when taken by a healthy person in allopathic doses is potentially of therapeutic value when administered in potentized form according to homeopathic principles. It follows, therefore, that the potential for new homeopathic remedies is limitless, and healthy volunteers must continue to be recruited. Although we now have over 3,000 homeopathic remedies available, we still tend to rely too much on the 200 or more classic remedies proved by Hahnemann and his co-workers.

Provings are the only way of identifying new homeopathic remedies which may be added to the *Materia Medica* and, as such, provings will always take up a major part of homeopathic research effort. With so many known but unproved plant species alone on this earth, the scope is enormous.

2. Proof of the Efficacy of Homeopathic Remedies

The dedicated homeopath accepts the fundamental truth of the basic precepts of Hahnemannian homeopathy and does not require proof of the effectiveness of homeopathic therapy other than the clinical evidence and his or her own experience.

After all, Hahnemann had dramatically demonstrated the effectiveness of homeopathic medicine in comparison with allopathic treatments in his time. After the Battle of Leipzig in 1813, Hahnemann's homeopathic treatment resulted in a mortality rate of little more than 1 percent against a high mortality rate among those patients receiving allopathic treatment. The cholera epidemic throughout Europe in the winter of 1831-32 and in Vienna in 1836, again gave Hahnemann the opportunity to demonstrate the superiority of homeopathic treatment. After Hahnemann's death, this success was repeated at the Royal London Homeopathic Hospital in England in 1854. During a cholera epidemic only 16.4 percent of patients in this hospital died, whereas 51.8 percent died in the allopathic hospitals (these results were deliberately suppressed by the medical establishment). Over the last century a mass of clinical evidence based on individual cases has been accumulated.

In modern times, much systematic research is conducted in this area, in part to improve the relative efficacy of homeopathic treatments, but more importantly to demonstrate to skeptical allopaths that, indeed, homeopathy does work. The latter aim is important if only because medical legislation in most countries (drawn up by allopaths) demands this proof, and in some countries is a precursor to the very survival of homeopathy. The problems in providing proof of efficacy in the context of allopathic protocols is discussed later in this chapter.

3. How Homeopathy Works

Although we have a broad understanding of the role of potencies in triggering or stimulating the body's own natural curative mechanism, we still have much to learn about *how* they trigger or stimulate the curative mechanism itself. Recent research, both allopathic and homeopathic, has thrown considerable light on this complex problem, for example, the AIDS epidemic which has sparked off much research into the nature of the body's immune system.

It must be stated that research into allopathic drugs relies heavily on clinical trials and relatively little is known of their curative processes. Dr. Blackie, the late physician to H.M. Queen Elizabeth of England, once remarked to a critical allopathic physician, "You tell me first how allopathic medicines work and I will tell you how ours work!"

4. Pharmacy Research

This area of research is important in assuring the integrity of the homeopathic medicines themselves, on which the physician relies for a successful practice. It is also crucial in ensuring that the medicines meet the legal requirements in each country where they are manufactured, particularly in relation to their quality. Nowadays, the larger manufacturers of homeopathic medicines are not only carrying out more and more research in this field, but they are also initiating and sponsoring significant research programs in the other clinical areas in hospitals and universities.

Although it is generally accepted that the rapid decline of homeopathy in the first half of the century was brought about largely by the onslaught of the so-called "miracle drug" revolution, the lack of research in homeopathy was another contributing factor. Homeopathy had become monolithic in character. Homeopaths of the day pointed to the enviable track records of 50 or more years of success in homeopathic treatment. As far as homeopathy was concerned, Hahnemann had said the last word. In fairness, however, it must be added that funds available for research were pathetically small—a problem which remains to the present day.

Hahnemann had written:

> The characteristic of novelty is in truth a capital crime in the orthodox school, which holds to its old doctrines and bends without reason under the yoke of methods consecrated only by time.

Hahnemann had in mind allopathic medicine, but his view, in the course of time, is equally valid of homeopathic doctrine itself. Dr. Max Tetau, in France, has stated the view that Hahnemann understood that youth was essential, and the survival of any medical doctrine relies on an atmosphere of contestation and perpetual renewal. Any medical discipline which is incapable of self criticism and which closes its doors to progress in modern science, and does not adapt them to its special philosophy, is condemned to disappear.

Dr. Nebel has commented that "Hahnemann gave us a skeleton but we must not ossify it."

Homeopathy must be dynamic and flexible, in a continuous state of evolution, and constantly alert to new medical and scientific developments if it is to grow in scope and stature. It must be stressed, however, that although new developments must be integrated into homeopathy, the fundamental Hahnemann concept of the Law of Similars and infinitesimal dilution in the context of a holistic approach are inviolable.

CRITERIA OF HOMEOPATHIC RESEARCH

As with any other field of medicine, homeopathy must, and can, demonstrate objective and undeniable evidence of its effectiveness. It will not suffice to rely on anecdotal evidence alone. Research is expensive and homeopathy has always been short of funds for this purpose. If only a fraction of the annual multi-million-dollar research expenditures for conventional medicine were made available to homeopathy, considerable progress could be made.

Professor Schofield of the University of London epitomized the critical allopathic view of the efficacy of homeopathic treatment:

> The homeopathic literature contains many reports of the successful use of remedies in the treatment of disease but, whereas these are no doubt of great value to the homeopath, the majority of reports are not of controlled trials and are of little value in making scientific assessment of the efficacy of homeopathy.

In most countries, the criteria for the approval of any allopathic or homeopathic medicine by the controlling bodies are:

1. Purity or quality.

The purity of homeopathic medicines can be guaranteed if they are prepared under a strict system of quality control described in Chapter 3. Quality control must include monitoring and testing at every stage of manufacture, from raw materials to the finished product. It is essential that those responsible are adequately trained and experienced. The finished medicine must be:

a. In compliance with the quality specifications.
b. Of the required purity.
c. Prepared in accordance with Hahnemann procedures.
d. Enclosed in a proper, sealed container.
e. Labeled correctly, including the potency.
f. Properly stored to ensure it retains its efficacy.

Homeopathic medicines which meet these criteria invariably meet legislative quality requirements in most countries.

2. *Safety. Non-toxic and free from dangerous side effects.*

The intrinsic safety of homeopathic treatment is accepted even by the most critical controlling bodies. We know that, by virtue of their high dilution, they are completely safe and non-addictive, with no unwanted side effects. There is no record of their rejection on this score in any country.

3. *Therapeutic effectiveness.*

Proof of the efficacy of specific homeopathic medicines relies on their undisputed track record of successful treatment for more than 175 years. Furthermore, if the fundamental principle of the Similimum is accepted, then it follows that the efficacy of the treatment must be accepted.

CLINICAL TRIALS

Criteria 1. and 2. above are, in the main, acceptable to the controlling bodies, but 3. is unacceptable, since only the conventional allopathic protocols of clinical evaluation are recognized. These are "double blind" or "double blind, crossover" clinical trials. The double-blind clinical trial is based on the premise that neither the physicians conducting the trial nor the patients undergoing the trial know which patients are being treated with the actual medicine or a placebo. In the crossover trial the medicine and placebo are interchanged at a given time in the period of the trial, without the knowledge of either doctor or patients.

A typical allopathic view was written in an article by M. M. Rouze in the French publication *Science et Vie*. He attacked homeopathy for failing to prove the effectiveness of its remedies and called for double-blind clinical studies, "which is the only true unequivocal test to which all *true* medicine must submit."

There are several reasons, however, which make it very difficult to reconcile homeopathic practice with protocols conceived solely for conventional medical treatment. These are as follows:

1. Homeopathic researchers have met with many obstructions from allopathic physicians for reasons of principle, expedience and a failure to understand homeopathic principles.

2. With the relatively small number of homeopathically treated patients, it is difficult to gather sufficient numbers suffering from the same disease to obtain statistically significant results.

3. Homeopathic treatment necessarily involves a long follow-up period, extending well beyond the usual limit of a clinical trial, to properly assess the benefit of the treatment.

4. The highly individualized nature of homeopathic treatment involves different treatment from one person to another for the same disease condition. That a homeopathic clinical trial necessarily requires a case-by-case study, that is, drug-symptoms-person is, in most cases, incompatible with the allopathic two-dimensional system of drug-symptoms. This extra dimension complicates the experimental design of any clinical trial enormously (see drawing).

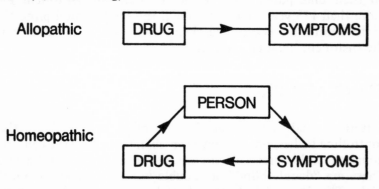

In 1981, with Drs. Jenkins and Campbell, I approached the Mathematics Research Center of the University of Warwick in England to discuss the feasibility of a three-dimensional clinical trial. After some research, they informed us that they could develop a mathematical model which would be appropriate at a cost of $500,000! The cost was a clear indication of the complexity of the problem.

Some controlled clinical trials have been carried out, however, treating carefully selected conditions. Others have employed homeopathic remedies which are near specific for the treatment of the chosen condition, in order to minimize the holistic dimension and reconcile the differences discussed above.

Probably the best controlled early blind clinical trial was conducted in 1944, in London and Glasgow, during World War II, by Dr. Paterson. It dealt with the prevention and treatment of mustard gas burns. Mustard Gas 30CH, Rhus Toxicodendron

30CH or other medicines were given to volunteers before and after applying mustard gas to the skin. The conclusions were that Rhus Toxicodendron 30CH given as a treatment, or Mustard Gas 30CH used prophylactically, resulted in a significant shift in the frequency of both deep and medium skin lesions with superficial lesions unaltered with the former medicine and an increase of superficial lesions with the latter. Reanalysis of the data in 1982 by Owen and Ives, using modern statistical methods, showed that the experiments did give unequivocal results in favor of Mustard Gas, Rhus Toxicodendron and Kali Bichromicum over placebos.

A successful double-blind clinical trial was conducted by Dr. P. Gibson et al. in 1978-1980, using a wide range of remedies to treat rheumatoid arthritis. Patients were treated with high doses of salicylate (44), individually prescribed homeopathic remedies (54) or a placebo (100). The results showed that patients treated homeopathically responded statistically better than those treated with salicylate or placebo, moreover they experienced no side effects. Criticism arose, however, since some of the patients treated homeopathically continued their previous allopathic treatment during the trial. A second, more rigidly controlled double-blind trial used a number of homeopathic remedies which were administered to suit individual patients, or placebo, to supplement conventional anti-inflammatory drugs.

Remedies were prescribed for each of the 46 patients taking part in the trial on an individual basis, according to classical homeopathic principles. To render the use of different remedies compatible with the protocols of a double-blind trial, a third party, acting independently without the knowledge of doctors or patients, arbitrarily split the patients between those receiving the prescribed remedy and those receiving the placebo. Progress or otherwise was monitored through the three-month period of the trial.

Results showed significant improvement in subjective pain, stiffness and grip strength in those patients receiving homeopathic remedies, whereas there was no significant change in those patients who received the placebo. These results showed that homeopathic treatment compared most favorably with conventional treatment. Furthermore, no side effects were reported.

In 1983, a double-blind, crossover clinical trial was conducted in London, jointly with homeopathic and allopathic physicians, to compare Rhus Toxicodendron 6x with an allopathic drug, Fenoprofen and a placebo in the treatment of osteoarthritis of the hip and knee. From the homeopathic point of view the results were unsatisfactory, in that Fenoprofen showed significant improvement over the placebo, whereas Rhus Toxicodendron showed no significant improvement in the patients' condition.

This trial was strongly criticized on several counts: the relatively small number of patients involved in the trial, the limited time of the trial—only two weeks and the use of Rhus Toxicodendron *only* on a limited symptom picture. Drs. Ghosh and Kennedy (1983) pointed out that acute conditions would have responded more rapidly to homeopathic treatment, whereas in chronic conditions constitutional remedies are most efficacious.

A single-blind trial, in 1976, to test the effect of Arnica on bruises found that, whereas Arnica 30CH had little effect in reducing bruising, Arnica 10M was very effective. The tests using Arnica 30CH involved the treatment of two consecutive trials on separate bruises. Again, it was difficult to assess the validity of the results as the trial was not conducted double-blind and lacked proper controls.

A single-blind trial conducted by Dr. P. Ustianowski in London in 1974 demonstrated the effectiveness of homeopathic treatment in comparison with the placebo response. In a sample of 200 women suffering from cystitis, 50 percent received a course of placebos and 50 percent received a course of Staphysagria 30CH. Ninety percent of those women treated with Staphysagria found complete relief of all symptoms within one month, while of those receiving the placebos only 40 percent lost all symptoms within one month.

An interesting controlled, randomized, double-blind trial studying the homeopathic treatment of migraine was conducted by Dr. B. Brigo et al. in Italy in 1986. Its aim was to assess the efficacy of homeopathic treatment compared with placebo in 60 patients suffering from migraine (30 patients treated with homeopathic remedies and 30 patients given placebo; 10 male and 50 female). One or two homeopathic remedies were selected from eight remedies—Belladonna, Cyclamen, Gelsemium, Ignatia, Lachesis, Natrum Muriaticum, Silica and Sulfur—given in single doses at 30CH potency. Types of migraine not presented in the characteristics of the chosen remedies were excluded. An exact diagnosis of the migraine was made in terms of frequency, periodicity, regularity, duration and concomitant symptoms for each patient.

A clinical examination of all patients was carried out during and two months after treatment. A final evaluation of the patients' response after four months demonstrated a significant reduction in the intensity and frequency of migraine in the patients treated with the homeopathic remedy.

	Placebo		Homeopathic Remedy	
Evaluation	No. of patients	%	No. of patients	%
Aggravation	1	3.3	0	0
No change	14	46.7	2	6.7
Insignificant improvement	6	20.0	0	0
Significant improvement	4	13.3	0	0
Quite good	1	3.3	4	13.3
Good	2	6.7	10	33.3
Very Good	2	6.7	14	46.7

This trial may be criticized on the basis of too few patients for the results to be statistically meaningful, and the use of more than one remedy.

Since 1983, the Boiron Institute in France (Dr. P. Belon et al.) has been presenting results of studies of the inhibition of basophil degranulation by Histaminum 7CH and Apis Mellifica 7CH in allergic patients. The double-blind trials consisted of performing a series of basophil degranulation tests, both in the presence of the homeopathic potency and in its absence. Histamine was chosen as it is known to be one of the main constituents of basophils. The effect of Apis Mellifica was studied in patients allergic to hymenopters. The controls were sterile, distilled water.

With Histaminum 7CH, 76 percent of the results were totally positive, 12 percent partially positive and only 12 percent were negative. Given the restricted number of blood samples with Apis Mellifica, results were difficult to assess. However, it was concluded that both Histaminum 7CH and Apis Mellifica 7CH have an anti-degranulating activity.

Subsequent studies (1987) were conducted on the activities of histamine dilutions on mite sensitized basophils, and the effect of dilutions of penicillin and aspirin on basophils sensitized to penicillin and aspirin. The conclusions were that 6CH and 7CH potencies of Histamine can inhibit basophil degranulation measured by the change of affinity of the granules for toluidine blue. It is believed that the inhibition by Histaminum 6CH is feasible if the hypothesis of an interference with the negative feedback of Histamine at the H2 receptor level is accepted. The effect of penicillin and aspirin potencies was shown to enhance both the effect of dilutions of the actual antigen and the specificity of the dilutions.

Other clinical trials, some of which have demonstrated the efficacy of homeopathic remedies, have suffered from lack of proper controls or results which were not statistically significant. But, in 1986, the results of a remarkably successful, randomized, double-blind, placebo-controlled clinical trial were published in *The Lancet*, under the title *"Is Homeopathy a Placebo Response? Controlled Trial of Homeopathic Potency, with Pollen in Hayfever as Model."* (D. Reilly, M. Taylor, C. McSharry, T. Aitchison). The study was carried out at the Glasgow Homeopathic Hospital in conjunction with Glasgow University's Department of Bacteriology and Immunology, the Western Infirmary and the University Department of Statistics. The effects of a 30CH potency of mixed grass pollen were compared with a placebo in 144 patients with active hayfever. The potency was prepared from 12 different species of grass most commonly associated with seasonal hayfever in the United Kingdom and administered in tablet form.

The conventional design of this clinical trial was made possible by a pilot study carried out by Reilly and Taylor in 1983, and earlier work on homeopathic allergen desensitization using house dust mite potencies by Drs. R.G. Gibson, S.L.M. Gibron, R.H. Harris-Owen and K. Datt-Lai.

Patients were selected from those who had suffered from seasonal rhinitis for a least two years and displayed current symptoms. Sufficient time had to have elapsed to eliminate the effects of any allopathic drugs taken by the patients. The patients received randomized Mixed Grass Pollen 30CH or placebo on a double-blind basis for two weeks to check for homeopathic aggravations and to give a base line for the study. Pollen counts were taken daily throughout the run-in period and the trial and symptom scores were adjusted on the basis of a computerized statistical analysis (see graphs on facing page).

The results proved conclusively that only the homeopathically treated group showed a clear reduction in symptoms. This difference was reflected in a reduced need for antihistamines (halving), an increased significance when adjusted for pollen count and time of season and by assessment of doctors. The response was most pronounced in the post-treatment period, suggesting that symptoms may have been aggravated unnecessarily by repetition of the dose. As expected, at least initially, aggravations were greater with those patients treated homeopathically.

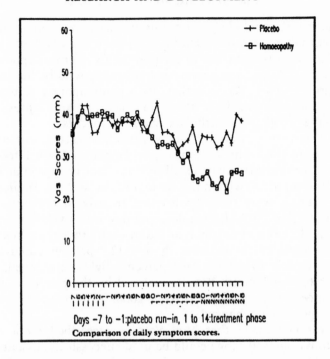

Days −7 to −1:placebo run-in, 1 to 14:treatment phase

Comparison of daily symptom scores.

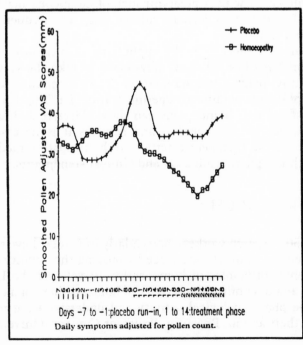

Days −7 to −1:placebo run-in, 1 to 14:treatment phase

Daily symptoms adjusted for pollen count.

The report concluded: *"The drug we used was potentized to the point where, in theory, none of the original material remained.* Yet these results and those of the pilot study offer no support for the suggestion that the observed effects were wholly due to the placebo responses. As such they are a contemporary statement of an empirical puzzle in its second century and represent a confusing challenge to orthodox scientific models."

An interesting study of Nux Vomica was carried out under the aegis of the Dolisos Company in France in 1983. Fifty-five patients, predominantly male, all showing multisymptomatology (6 to 10 symptoms) within the context of the *Materia Medica* for Nux Vomica, were treated with this remedy in potencies between 3CH and 30CH. One dose per day was given for two to eight weeks, sometimes in association with other remedies. Results assessed by the patients showed 12.7 percent cured; 67.3 percent greatly improved; 16.4 percent slightly improved; and 3.6 percent unchanged. Results assessed by the physician were 29.4 percent very good; 49 percent good; 18 percent moderate; and 3.6 percent unchanged.

It was concluded that Nux Vomica prescribed for a wide symptomatological range could be used successfully, essentially in chronic cases with a predominance of cutaneous manifestations indicative of underlying allergy and, less frequently, in acute conditions.

The limited success in the application of orthodox clinical trial procedures has led many physicians to take the view that homeopathy, being a unique medical practice, requires its own specific protocols of clinical experimentation. Dr. Tetau et al., in France, stated that homeopathy can show objective and undeniable evidence of effectiveness, and believes it is necessary to demonstrate the therapeutic activity of homeopathic medicines from both the pharmacological and clinical standpoints.

BASIC RESEARCH

Since 1950, research workers, particularly in France, have striven to supplement clinical experience by proving the validity of the fundamental principles of homeopathy, to validate the Law of Similars and to confirm the activity of homeopathic potencies; to prove the pharmacological activity and understand the mechanism of their action. Recently, Professor Camber (University of

Bordeaux) et al. have demonstrated the protective effect of potencies of mercury and cadmium in relation to substances toxic to the kidneys. In Montpelier, Professor Bastide et al. have studied the relationship between homeopathic potencies and the immunological system. A paper on the immune modulation of potencies of Thymusinum or of its derivative hormones was published in 1982. Professor Narcisse of the University of Tours has carried out research studies aimed toward the mechanism of action in relation to the idea of receptors. The importance of receptors is well recognized in contemporary pharmacology. They play a vital role in the transmission of information at the cellular level and more generally in the regulation of human behavior.

Following the work in the United States by Dr. Bourne et al., Professor Narcisse has demonstrated the activity of homeopathic potencies of Histaminum. In the last 25 years, in seeking to demonstrate the activity of homeopathic potencies, considerable attention has been given to the effect of homeopathic potencies on the growth of plants. It is believed that they replaced missing trace elements or deficiencies in trace elements.

In 1966, Dr. Netien reported on the effect of Cuprum Sulfuricum 15CH on plants poisoned by solutions of copper sulfate. Dr. P. Koffler (1965) and Dr. W. Annamaker (1968) published work on the effect of potencies of sulfur and boron on the growth of onions. Annamaker claimed that the weight and length of plants as well as their mineral content was affected by treating the soil with sulfur and boron potencies, while Koffler demonstrated considerable differences in the growth and sulfur content of seedlings grown in soil treated with potencies of sulfur, compared with placebo treatment.

Dr. W. Boyd, in Scotland, reported in 1954 on the biological and biochemical evidence of the activity of Mercurius Muriaticum 30CH on starch-diastase preparations. In France, Dr. Heintz measured the behavioral pattern of fish and other animals in response to different potencies.

Subsequently, Drs. Pelikan and Unger (1971) studied the effect of potencies of Argentum Nitricum on the growth of wheat seedlings. In a series of growth experiments, repeated six times, they found that each series gave the same growth curve pattern of stimulated growth rate for potencies of 8x and higher. Dr. Basold had carried out similar experiments in 1968, and claimed significant increases in growth rates of wheat seedlings using Argenticum Nitricum potencies, but his results did not stand up to statistical analysis.

Drs. Jones and Jenkins carried out similar studies at the Royal London Homeopathic Hospital in England in 1981, using centesimal potencies of Argenticum Nitricum, Arnica Montana and several other substances and found similar curves of increasing in mean growth rates with increasing potency (see graph). In 1983, they used wheat and yeast, tested with an improved experimental technique. Using centesimal potencies of Pulsatilla, they found that some potencies stimulated growth while others inhibited growth. The mean extension growth curves indicated potencies of optimum activity generally in line with those potencies most commonly prescribed in practice. Dr. Steffen repeated this work in 1983.

In 1967, Dr. Netien et al. performed experiments in the treatment of experimental diabetes with mice. Again in France in 1976, Dr. Aubin et al. studied the action of different potencies of phosphorus on the livers of rats. In 1981, at the Marie Curie Institute in London, the lead content of the urine of rats and mice when treated with Plumbum Metallicum 200CH showed excretion levels comparable to the conventional treatment with penicillins. The use of animals in these experiments was severely criticized by many homeopaths, particularly as they could have been carried out, quite safely, with human volunteers.

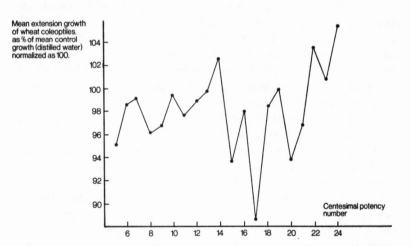

Graph of extension growth vs. potency for centesimal dilutions of Arnica Montana.

Reference: Jenkins and Jones, Royal Homeopathic Hospital.

Interferons

The isolation and identification of the interferons during the 1980s has been observed by homeopathic physicians with considerable interest. These organic substances—polypeptides—are produced in human blood cells, in minute quantities, in response to the attack on the blood cells by a disease virus. On passing into the plasma the interferons are believed to destroy the disease virus. Several types of interferon have now been identified. This demonstration of the body's natural defense system, recognized by the allopaths, is entirely compatible with homeopathic principles. Interferon is "manufactured" outside the human body by treating blood cells contained in a thermostatically controlled vessel with a disease virus (for example, a particular strain of influenza) to cause the blood cells to produce interferons, which are extracted continuously in very small quantities over a period of up to 36 hours. The interferon thus produced is administered to patients in allopathic doses to supplement their body's own natural supply, thus speeding their recovery. Enormously expensive, allopathic doses have given encouraging results with certain forms of cancer.

In 1980, the author attempted to set up a research program to study the effect of homeopathic potencies introduced into the production system described above. If such experiments had shown that the added homeopathic potency catalyzed, that is, increased the rate of formation of interferons in the system, then it could have provided knowledge of not only how homeopathy works, but also incontrovertible proof that it does work. Regrettably, the allopathic manufacturing laboratories refused to cooperate. A pilot experiment was carried out at the University of California in 1981 and a positive result was obtained, but the details were not published.

Computers

Since 1977, considerable research effort has been directed in the application of computers in homeopathy. Computers are now commonly used for the storage of patient histories. Work is proceeding in the United States to build a comprehensive computer data base, and several computerized Repertories are now being marketed in the United States and Europe.

Biotherapies

In 1964, homeopathic physicians in France developed a new branch of homeopathy known as Biotherapy. Biotherapy comprises Organotherapy, Gemmotherapy and Lithotherapy.

Organotherapy

Homeopathic potencies of healthy glands or tissues are called sarcodes. Dr. Conan first introduced glandular extracts in his range of homeopathic remedies. This was followed by Dr. Nebel et al. in Lausanne and Drs. Fortier-Bernoville, Martiny and Rouy in 1936. In recent years, extensive research by Drs. Tetau, Guermondrez, Gogmos, Bergeret and Professor Bastide of Montpellier has been carried out to evaluate Organotherapy on a wide scale. Detailed reference to these studies was published by Drs. Tetau and Bergeret (*L'Organothérapie Diluée et Dynamisée*). A complete list of sarcodes is given in Appendix 3.

Organotherapy is defined as a form of homeopathic treatment used in various glands of the human body in order to rectify disturbed function, and involving the administration of homologous glandular and tissue extracts prepared according to Hahnemman's procedure.

Organs are removed under veterinary supervision from healthy pigs, cattle or sheep. The organs are subsequently frozen in dry ice, transported and converted into the remedies. The strains have truly synergistic effects aimed at acting upon the whole organ. For example, cartilage is taken from different joints, from the largest to the smallest, at the site of insertion of the ligaments; colon mucosa is taken at different levels within the colon.

Organotherapy does not aim for a substitutive or palliative effect, but a direct action on the gland or tissue involved, restoring its disturbed function by stimulation or reduction in a precise manner.

One of the essential concepts of Organotherapy is cellular specificity, glandular or tissular. Thus, *the organ acts upon the organ*. The diseased organ is selectively sensitive to its healthy homologue. For example, the intestine may be treated with intestinal extracts by an immunopathological mechanism.

The second principle of Organotherapy is concerned with the potencies administered, or the triphasic activity of the medication.

Hence: Low potencies of organs—4CH and 5CH—are stimulant. Medium potencies of organs—7CH—are regulatory. High potencies of organs—9CH, 12CH and 30CH—are depressant. For example, Folliculinum 4CH stimulates ovarian section of Folliculine and Thyrodia 4CH stimulates thyroid secretion. Higher potencies of 9CH, 12CH and 30CH inhibit secretion of the corresponding glands.

This phenomenon has been demonstrated experimentally. Each living organ is capable of recognizing its own substance. This tissue "memory" ensures identical multiplication of cells. Patients in whom Organotherapy is used are suffering from auto-immune conflict, which has been proved biologically. Organotherapy, therefore, provides a further demonstration of the interrelationship between homeopathy and immunology. Administration of organotherapeutic medicaments is said to produce immune tolerance.

According to Dr. Max Tetau, Organotherapy in low potencies results in an overwhelming antigenic effect which frees the organ and thereby stimulates its function as the production of anti-organ antibodies is interrupted. Another explanation may be that within damaged tissues there are toxic complex substances (reagins) consisting of the union of anti-organ bodies with the antigen represented by the tissue itself in the process of recovery. The organotherapeutic medication is a specific antigen which substitutes itself for the damaged tissue antigen and combines with the anti-organ antibodies, forming a new complex which replaces the toxic complex. Normal function of the organ is, therefore, restored and hence stimulated.

Organotherapeutic medicines are administered as granules or liquid. The standard dose is 5 granules (pills) dissolved under the tongue or 10 drops of liquid on the tongue using a glass dropper. It should not be administered too frequently—three times a week is the usual frequency. In certain acute cases, daily doses may be prescribed.

Examples of organotherapeutic treatment are as follows:

Depression

Hypothalamus 7CH, first evening. Cerebrinum 7CH, second evening.

Thyroid Regulation

Thyrodia 7CH, three doses per week.

Premenstrual Syndrome

Folliculinum 9CH, seventh and twenty-first day of cycle.

Influenza

Adrenal Cortex (Corticosurrenale) 4CH, three times a week.

Anemia

Bone Marrow (Meduloss) 7CH, first evening. Spleen (Splenine) 7CH, second evening.

It must be noted that there is some variability of the clinical activity or Organotherapy potencies in relation to the individual sensitivity of the patient.

Gemmotherapy

This branch of biotherapy was originally introduced in France by Dr. Henry and, since 1965, has been developed clinically by Dr. Tetau. Gemmotherapy employs potencies of the buds of fresh plants or embryonic tissues in the growth phase, such as young shoots. These tissues are rich in growth factors, including hormones, auxins and gibberellins. Today, homeopathic medication can offer more than 40 Gemmotherapy preparations, which opens up an exciting new field.

These preparations are prepared according to the French Pharmacopoeia by maceration of the fresh buds or shoots in alcoholized glycerine and, after filtration, potentized in the second decimal strength according to Hahnemannian procedures. Only this dilution is used by homeopathic physicians at the present time, although it is likely that further research will reveal other optimum potencies.

Given the affinity each of the buds presents for each of the organs of the human body, it is possible to give specific clinical indications. Thus, we have Ribes Nigrum (Black Currant buds), an outstanding Gemmotherapy preparation, rich in vitamin C, anthocyanins and flavonoids. All of these active principles are well known for their anti-inflammatory properties, which act on the microcirculation. Ribes Nigrum is truly an outstanding preparation; the Black Currant bud has a marked analgesic effect on all pneumonia.

Other examples of Gemmotherapy are buds of Pinus Montana (Mountain Pine), which has a eutrophic effect on articular cartilage; buds of Vitis Vinifera (Grape Vine), which regulates bone metabolism and inhibits proliferation deformaties; and buds of Sequoia Gigantea, an excellent anti-senescent substance for the elderly man. Dr. Tetau has described Gemmotherapy as a modern form of homeopathic drainage which opens up the possibility of true tissue potentization therapy.

The most frequently used dose is 50 to 70 drops per day of 2x potency for up to two months' duration.

Some other Gemmotherapy medications with their indications are given below:

Abies Pectinata (Firbuds)—Decalcification, alvedo-dental pyorrhea.

Betula Verrucosa (Birch seeds)—Intellectual overwork.

Carpinus Betulus (Hornbeam buds)—Bronchitis, spasmodic cough.

Cedrus Libani (Young shoots of cedar)—Dry eczema, pruritus.

Crataegus Oxycantha (Hawthorne buds)—Tachycardia.

Fraxinus Excelsior (Ash buds)—Gout.

Juniperus Communis (Young shoots of Juniper)—Cirrhosis.

Rose Canina (dogrose buds)—Headache, migraine.

Tilia Tomentosa (Lime tree buds)—Neuralgia, neurotic conditions, nervous sedative, insomnia.

Viburnum Lantana (Viburnum buds)—Asthma.

Lithotherapy

Lithotherapy was developed by Drs. Tetau and Bergeret in France. It employs potencies prepared from selected natural minerals and rocks to reestablish trace metallic or metalloidic balances of the organism.

The importance of trace elements in the body, such as copper, cobalt and manganese, in the activity of some enzymes is now known. Certain illnesses, however, are based theoretically on the deficiency of metallic ions, although the body content of these ions is quite normal. For example, in osteoporosis, the calcium-phosphorus balance is often quite normal. It would appear that the organism cannot utilize these ions because of some kind of blockage. This "blockage" is due to the chemical process of *chelation*, in which the metal acceptor atom receives a number of shared pairs of electrons from an organic compound. The metal is gripped in the "claws" of the organic molecule (hence,

the name chelation from the Greek *chele,* the claw of a crab),
and is effectively removed from active metabolism.
A typical chelation may be illustrated thus:

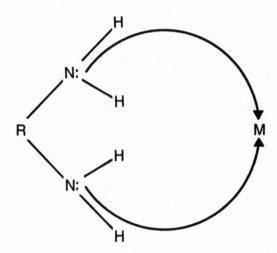

Where R = an organic grouping containing one or more
carbon atoms, N = Nitrogen atom (donor), M = metal atom
(acceptor) and : are pairs of electrons.

The excretion of arsenic in animals was studied by Drs.
Wurmser and Lapp in 1935, after dosing with Arsenicum Album
7CH, when it was demonstrated that the homeopathic potency
was capable of releasing the blocked arsenic.

Lithotherapy employs potencies of naturally occurring rocks
and minerals consisting of complex crystalline, inorganic structures. These crystalline structures are analogous to chelated
compounds and can liberate metallic ions. In practice, potencies
of 8x are found to be most efficacious.

Indications of Lithotherapeutic Substances

Mineral	Principal Constituents	Indications
Native Silver	Silver	Analgesic, anti-inflammatory
Apatite	Calcium, Fluorine, phosphorus	Inflammatory rheumatism
Bornite	Copper, iron	Anti-inflammatory agent
Chalcopyrites	Copper, iron	Inflammatory rheumatism

Conglomerate	Silicon	Dry and weeping eczema
Barytine	Barium	Vertigo
Galena	Lead	All types of allergy
Garnierite	Nickel	Disorders of pancreatic endocrine function
Pink Sandstone	Silicon	Constipation
Iron Pyrites	Iron, sulfur	Vesticular pains
Hematite	Iron	Anemia
Lazulite	Aluminon, iron, magnesium	Cramp in lower limbs
Lepidolite	Lithium, aluminon, iron	Depressive states
Pyrolusite	Manganese	All types of allergy
Rhodonite	Manganese, silicon	Insomnia

PHARMACEUTICAL RESEARCH AND DEVELOPMENT

The strict procedures for the preparation of the remedies laid down by Hahnemann in the *Organon* were scientifically sound and, apart from the occasional use of the Korsakovian method of potentization since 1832, for higher potencies, is still valid to the present day. Research and development in recent years, however, in techniques of medication, quality control and the scientific study of potencies has made significant progress using modern scientific knowledge and sophisticated instruments not available to Hahnemann.

Medication Techniques

Samples of placebo tablets impregnated with homeopathic medicament by hand methods have been shown, by the application of starch-iodide coloration tests, to have not been fully impregnated. In 1982, the Dolisos laboratories in France innovated a new process for perfecting the complete impregnation of placebo granules with the homeopathic medicament. The process, which differs from the classic technique of sugar coating of the granules, achieves a coefficient of impregnation of nearly 100 percent throughout the bulk, and achieves a much more significant absorption capacity of the homeopathic potencies.

Quality Control

New quality control procedures have considerably improved the purity and reliability of the finished medicines. Analytical techniques and testing equipment, including infrared spectroscopy, nuclear magnetic resonance spectroscopy, spectrophotometers, pH meters and refractometers, have raised standards of quality extensively in recent years and providing favorable comparison with the quality of conventional pharmaceutical manufacture.

Thin layer chromatography techniques (see Chapter 3) have been optimized in the analysis of mother tinctures. With the accuracy achieved, it is now possible to identify not only different mother tinctures, but also to identify the same mother tincture produced in different batches.

Microcrystallization

This technique was developed in 1976, and provides a means of identification of mother tinctures. Tests are performed by making a balanced mixture of nickel or chromium salts and a mother tincture. The mixture is then crystallized under controlled conditions of humidity and temperature, and the resultant crystal pattern viewed or photographed under a microscope using a special filter system. Each mother tincture produces a distinctive crystalline pattern of organo-metallic salts, which can be compared with a standard pattern. This technique is not feasible with liquid potencies, but it provides a spectacular illustration of the variety, the natural beauty, and complexity of homeopathic medicines.

THE NATURE OF POTENCIES

The paradox of the effective microdose, whereby potencies may contain only molecules of the diluent alcohol and water above the Avogadro limit, has stimulated considerable research over the last 50 years. Much of the work has been directed towards identifying physical and chemical differences between high potencies and solutions of pure ethyl alcohol and water.

Reports of significant differences in conductivity, refractive indices and dipole moments are unsubstantiated. It has been suggested that the potentization procedure, particularly the succussion step, induces different electronic configurations or electrochemical patterning in the solution (G.P. Barnard and J.H. Stevenson, U.S.A., 1967). These patterns or configurations are assumed to be replicated at each successive potentization far beyond the dilution, where theoretically none of the original molecules of mother tincture exist. Thus the "thumbprint" of the original substance is carried through to the very highest potencies. R.L. Jones and M.D. Jenkins (U.K., 1983) demonstrated that changes in the effect of potencies on yeast growth was dependent on the succussion procedure. It has also been suggested by P. Callinan in 1985 that succussion stores potential energy in the bonds of the alcohol/water solution which can be demonstrated in the infrared spectrum. W.E. Boyd has suggested a biophysical rather than a biochemical model would be more appropriate in determining the nature of potencies.

Nuclear magnetic resonance (NMR) studies of succussed solutions have proved fruitful. T.M. Young (U.S.A., 1975) provided evidence that resonance images distinguished between succussed solutions and simple dilutions. Studies in Holland (*Science of The Total Environment*, 1987) claimed to have demonstrated some type of sub-atomic activity in potencies higher than 24X, above the Avogadro limit. It was reported that this work was being taken up by Dr. Om Ganda at Harvard Medical School.

THE FUTURE OF HOMEOPATHY

In view of the sustained prejudiced and bigoted opposition to homeopathy throughout the world for nearly 180 years, it is unrealistic to suppose that homeopathy will show more than a marginal increase in its acceptance by the medical establishment in the foreseeable future. Homeopathy will not be wholly accepted until it is included in the syllabuses of the university medical schools at undergraduate level, since its omission leads to inevitable prejudice of generations of physicians. Some day it is hoped that University Professorships may be established and the case for homeopathy may be heard.

The marked increase in public demand for homeopathic treatment over the last ten years has not peaked yet. A survey in the United Kingdom, carried out in 1984 by the Institute of Complementary Medicine, showed that the number of people consulting homeopathic practitioners was increasing by 15 to 20 percent annually. One million people were receiving homeopathic treatment (about 2 percent of the population). In the United States in 1986, it was estimated that approximately the same number of people were treated homeopathically (about 0.4 percent of the population), with a similar growth rate. In France, where homeopathy is particularly strong, it is estimated that almost 20 percent of the population has turned to homeopathy.

The use of homeopathy in conjunction with other holistic therapies, such as acupuncture, osteopathy, chiropractic and herbal medicine, will become more commonplace. The number of multi-therapy clinics will expand considerably. This trend is particularly marked in the United States.

Homeopathy is now generally regarded as a complementary medicine to conventional medicine, rather than an alternative medicine, which is an encouraging trend, since this concept reduces the conflict between the two therapies. Increasing leisure time in a more affluent society will continue to increase health consciousness, manifested by the trend towards natural foods, proper dieting, regular exercise and a recognition of the dangers of environmental pollution. This is entirely in accord with the homeopathic approach to health as a natural, safe therapy and it will be a significant factor in its growth in the future.

Homeopathy, not unnaturally, attracts people who are individualists—free thinking, sensitive people with strong convictions—like Samuel Hahnemann himself. While these are admirable qualities, it leads inevitably to divisions and conflict within homeopathy itself. Divisions arise between physicians with conflicting views on different aspects of homeopathy, for example, the division between the high-potency "Kentists" and the low-potency "Hughesians." Further differences prevalent among lay supporters of homeopathy in most countries have led to the division and subdivision of many lay groups and societies. As long as homeopathy enjoys the support of only a small minority, these divisions inevitably weaken homeopathy. It is to be hoped that in the course of time, these organizations will gradually come together again as unified bodies, presenting a common united front to those who oppose homeopathy, surely a classic example of the old adage, "United we stand, divided we fall."

As the world becomes smaller through modern travel and better communications, there will be a closer cooperation between homeopaths worldwide. This partnership of people with a common bond will do much to solve the common problems facing homeopathy in more than 60 countries. International bodies, such as the International Homeopathic Medical League (Liga Medicorum Homeopathica Internationalis) and the International Association of Homeopathic Veterinary Surgeons will flourish.

Money must be found to fund extensive scientific and medical research into every facet of homeopathy. At the present time, only the few larger companies manufacturing homeopathic medicines can afford to engage in homeopathic research. The scope for such research is vast; the greatest fillip to the acceptance of homeopathy could come through a breakthrough in the cure of diseases hitherto incurable, such as certain forms of cancer, heart disease and AIDS.

Much more research must be carried out in proving new homeopathic medicines, which is the only valid method. Relatively few new medicines have been added to the *Homeopathic Materia Medica* this century. It is with some humility that we must acknowledge the fact that only five to ten percent of over half a million known plant species on this earth have been studied for the homeopathic curative potential. Research is expensive. More money must be found to fund homeopathic research.

Furthermore, we still (like the allopaths) have only a limited understanding as to how homeopathy works. Indeed, in spite of all modern scientific and medical progress in this century, we are, metaphorically, groping in the early morning mists of a single day in almost two centuries of homeopathic progress. I hope our successors will view our present understanding and knowledge in this way, as homeopathy will have achieved its great potential for the relief of suffering mankind.

The author would like to leave the last words to Dr. Samuel Hahnemann himself. Expressing his own sentiments in a letter from Leipzig to his dear friend Dr. Stapf in September 1815, he wrote:

> At present homeopathy grows with slow progress amid the abundance of weeds which luxuriate about it. It grows unobserved, from an unlikely acorn into a little plant; soon its head may be seen overtopping the tall weeds. Be patient—it is striking roots deep into the earth; it is strengthening it-

self unperceived, but all the more certainly in its own time it will increase, until it becomes an oak of God, whose arms stretch so that the suffering children of men may be revived under its beneficent shadow.

6 HOMEOPATHIC TREATMENT

FIFTY COMMON HOMEOPATHIC REMEDIES

1. Aconitum Napellus
2. Actaea Racemosa
3. Apis Mellifica
4. Argentum Nitricum
5. Arnica Montana
6. Arsenicum Album
7. Atropa Belladonna
8. Berberis Vulgaris
9. Bryonia Alba
10. Calcarea Carbonica
11. Calcarea Fluorica
12. Calcarea Phosphorica
13. Calendula Officinalis
14. Cantharis Vesicatoria
15. Carbo Vegetabilis
16. Chamomilla
17. Chelidonium Majus
18. Colchicum Autumnale
19. Cuprum Metallicum
20. Drosera Rotundifolia
21. Euphrasia Officinalis
22. Ferrum Phosphoricum
23. Gelsemium Sempervirens
24. Graphites
25. Hamamelis Virginiana
26. Hepar Sulfuris
27. Hydrastis Canadensis
28. Hypericum Perforatum
29. Ignatia Amara
30. Ipecacuanha
31. Kali Bichromicum
32. Kali Phosphoricum
33. Lachesis Mutus
34. Ledum Palustre
35. Lycopodium Clavatum
36. Magnesium Phosphoricum
37. Mercurius Vivus
38. Natrum Muriaticum
39. Nux Vomica
40. Phosphorus
41. Phytolacca Decandra
42. Pulsatilla Nigricans
43. Rhus Toxicodendron
44. Ruta Graveolens
45. Sepia Officinalis
46. Silica
47. Sulfur
48. Symphytum Officinalis
49. Thuja Occidentalis
50. Urtica Urens

SELECTING THE REMEDIES

In the table which follows, many common ailments and conditions are listed in alphabetical order. Symptoms, associated symptoms and sensations are listed for each condition, together with constitutional factors and modalities.

119

The appropriate remedies are listed on the right hand side of the page. These remedies most closely match the symptoms, modalities and constitution of the patient. It must be emphasized that a perfect match is rarely found, but the remedy giving the closest match of all the factors considered generally proves to be the most effective. The next closest match could be considered as a follow-up, or an alternative remedy.

Some remedies are near-specific in the treatment of a particular ailment and will prove effective in most cases. These remedies are printed in italics.

To quote J.H. Clarke, "the absence of any particular characteristic of a remedy is not contra-indication of its use provided other indications are sufficiently pronounced."

It has been necessary to restrict the choice to 50 common homeopathic remedies and polychrests only. Furthermore, the constitutional factors and modalities listed are not exhaustive. The reader is urged to consult the *Homeopathic Materia Medica* for detailed information on the full range of remedies available.

The table has been drawn up by reference to nine major homeopathic works, representing a complete library of clinical experience.

Dosages are given in Chapter 4. For the ailments listed, a potency of 12x or 6CH is recommended, although the correct choice of remedy is more likely to prove beneficial to the patient for acute conditions than the choice of potency.

Government regulations call for a warning with all medicines that, for pregnant women or those nursing a baby, the advice of a qualified health professional should be sought.

All medicines must be kept out of the reach of children.

To illustrate the use of the following tables, two examples are given:

Example 1

	Possible Remedies
BILIOUS ATTACK	Bryonia Alba
	Nux Vomica
	Berberis
	Chelidonium Majus
—with constipation and depression	Bryonia Alba
	Nux Vomica
	Berberis
—dark hair and complexion	Bryonia Alba
	Nux Vomica
—better in the evening —irritable person	*Nux Vomica*

Example 2

	Possible Remedies
CATARRH	Kali Bichromicum
	Calcarea Fluorica
	Euphrasia Officinalis
	Natrum Muriaticum
	Graphites
	Pulsatilla Nigricans
—yellowish discharge	Kali Bichromicum
	Calcarea Fluorica
	Pulsatilla Nigricans
—worse between 4 a.m. and 5 a.m.	
—stringy catarrh	*Kali Bichromicum*

Symptoms/Sensations	Constitutions/Modalities	Remedies
ABDOMEN, DISTENDED		
	Fat children.	CALCAREA CARBONICA
Hard; bloated; cold feeling.	Slim, rickety, obstinate children. Better for heat. Worse in morning and drinking alcohol.	SILICA
With flatulence; great pain.	Worse between 4 and 6 p.m.	LYCOPODIUM CLAVATUM
With hysteria; rumbling in bowels; throbbing pain in abdomen.	Worse in the morning, after meals, drinking coffee. Better while eating.	IGNATIA AMARA
Sensation of a living animal inside abdomen.	Worse before 3 a.m.	THUJA OCCIDENTALIS
With offensive flatulence; sharp thrusts through abdomen.	Worse from least touch or motion. Better lying down.	ARNICA MONTANA
ABDOMINAL PAINS		
Aching, dull pain.	Improves after resting.	ARNICA MONTANA
Food lies like a stone in stomach. When coughing.	Worse about 3 a.m.	BRYONIA ALBA
With flatulence; bloated feeling after meals; constipation.	Worse in afternoon, particularly 4 to 8 p.m. Better for warm applications and by motion	LYCOPODIUM CLAVATUM
Flatulence and colic after overeating and alcohol.	Dark, irritable persons. Worse for movement	NUX VOMICA

Symptoms/Sensations	Constitutions/Modalities	Remedies
Abdomen sensitive and painful; sensitive in liver region.	Worse after sleep. Better warm applications. Sensitive to clothing around waist.	LACHESIS MUTUS
	Before or during periods. Worse about 4 p.m.	PULSATILLA NIGRICANS
After vomiting.	Worse for pressure and drinking alcohol.	LACHESIS MUTUS

ABSCESSES

With redness, pain, and throbbing; little swelling; skin is hot and sensitive.	Worse about 3 p.m. Worse for cold.	ATROPA BELLADONNA
Much swelling; with or without pain; pinkness or redness; throbbing; intradermisedema.	Worse for warmth. Better for cold and in open air.	APIS MELLIFICA
Slow to mature; sensitive to touch; at beginning of suppuration.	Worse for cold. Better for warmth.	HEPAR SULFURIS
Mouth abscesses; thirst; moist mouth.	Worse at night, lying on right side.	MERCURIUS VIVUS
With suppuration and slow to clear; near rectum; after breakage to drain the pus.	Better for warmth. Worse for cold and humid weather.	SILICA
Abscess of the breast; pale breast; hardening beginning.	Worse by movement.	BRYONIA ALBA

ACIDITY

Belching; flatulence; radiating pain; from anxiety over coming event.	Worse for warmth, cold food, candies. Better for pressure.	ARGENTUM NITRICUM
After overeating and drinking.	Aversion to acid and cold foods. Worse before 3 a.m.	NUX VOMICA
Severe heartburn; bitter taste in mouth.	Worse from cold food and from 4 p.m. to 8 p.m. Better for motion and after midnight and warmth.	LYCOPODIUM CLAVATUM

ACNE

	Full-blooded, red-faced persons.	ATROPA BELLADONNA
With prominent pustules; bleed easily.	Particularly in youths.	HEPAR SULFURIS

Symptoms/Sensations	Constitutions/Modalities	Remedies
	Pale, weepy persons with fair hair.	PULSATILLA NIGRICANS
With scarring; throbbing; red face.	Slim, obstinate young people. Worse in morning, from washing and cold. Better from warmth.	SILICA
Simple acne.	Young persons.	CARBO VEGETABILIS

ACNE ROSACEA

From overdrinking, especially alcohol.	Slim, active, nervous, dark complexioned people.	NUX VOMICA
	Full-blooded, red-faced persons.	ATROPA BELLADONNA
Shiny, red, swollen nose.	Better from heat.	RHUS TOXICODENDRON
Burning sensations; itching, scaly.	Worse from cold, wet weather and scratching. Better from heat.	ARSENICUM ALBUM
Juvenile acne; hard symmetric pustules.	Worse from touch.	ARNICA MONTANA

ADENOIDS

	Pale, overweight children. Cold feet. Perspiring of head at night.	CALCAREA CARBONICA
	Children with persistent hunger, especially at 11 a.m.	SULFUR
Large, troublesome adenoids.	Slim, anemic, dark-complected children.	CALCAREA PHOSPHORICA

AGGRESSIVENESS

Sudden and violent.	Worse about 3 p.m.	ATROPA BELLADONNA
From mental strain; reproaching others.	Slim, easily offended persons, with tendency to headaches and dyspepsia.	NUX VOMICA
Occasional.	Sometimes depressed and apathetic.	SEPIA OFFICINALIS

ALCOHOLISM

With restlessness and mental disturbance; unquenchable thirst; exhaustion; loss of weight.	Better for warmth and warm drinks. Worse from food and after midnight.	ARSENICUM ALBUM
Hangovers, morning vomiting, tremulousness.	Dark complected, irritable persons. Worse before 3 a.m.	NUX VOMICA

Symptoms/Sensations	Constitutions/Modalities	Remedies
With fear and delirium.	Worse from tobacco smoke and in evening before midnight.	ACONITUM NAPELLUS
To relieve craving and withdrawal symptoms.	Worse about 11 a.m.	SULFUR
Frequently drunk.	Loud, voluble persons preferring company when overdrinking.	LACHESIS MUTUS

ANAL DISORDERS

Bleeding from difficult stool; anus sore and raw; bleeding hemorrhoids.	Worse in moist, warm air.	HAMAMELIS VIRGINIANA
Bleeding or itching with prolapse of anus.	Worse at night, on getting warm in bed, and washing.	SULFUR
Itching; burning.	Dark complected persons. Worse before 3 a.m. Better for lying down.	NUX VOMICA
Ready bleeding; with protrusion; moisture about anus; cramping.	Worse for physical exertion, change of weather and in evening.	PHOSPHORUS
Protruding piles; soreness; itching, blue suppurating; offensive; itching	Worse from cold and at night and 4 to 5 p.m.	CARBO VEGETABILIS
Piles with pressure and soreness in anus and rectum; itching and stitching up rectum; painful constriction of anus after stool.	Moody people. Worse for fresh air, sitting and standing, and in the morning. Better while walking.	IGNATIA AMARA
Bleeding piles with much pain. Burning in rectum.	Worse in cold, damp weather, from touch or exposure.	HYPERICUM PERFORATUM
Fissure with piles. (See HEMORRHOIDS)	Worse at 9 a.m.	CHAMOMILLA

ANGER

Arising from fright; for example, a near accident.	Worse in evening and at night and from music.	ACONITUM NAPELLUS
	Fractious children or cantankerous behavior of elderly persons. Worse for warmth.	CHAMOMILLA
Easily aroused at slightest cause; ferocious.	With rapid speech. Blonde people. Worse for cold.	HEPAR SULFURIS

Symptoms/Sensations	Constitutions/Modalities	Remedies
ANGINA PECTORIS		
Pseudo or imagined angina, caused by wind or overeating.	Particularly 4 to 5 p.m.	CARBO VEGETABILIS
ANKLES, SWOLLEN		
Simple swelling; stinging pain.	Worse for heat or touch and 4 to 6 p.m. Better for cold bathing.	APIS MELLIFICA
From varicose veins.		HAMAMELIS VIRGINIANA
With rheumatic pain: cold, clammy legs at night.	Worse at night and wet, damp weather.	MERCURIUS VIVUS
ANXIETY		
With rheumatic and hysterical symptoms; depression; fear of death.	Especially women.	ACTAEA RACEMOSA
Worried about the future; suicidal tendency; nightmares; restlessness.	Worse in the evening and after midnight and after drinking.	DROSERA ROTUNDIFOLIA
Fear of disease, sudden misfortune, or death; despair of life; cold extremities.	Pale, flabby, sweaty persons. Worse about 2 p.m.	CALCAREA CARBONICA
After shock or fright; sudden onset of anxiety of panic; from fear.	Better in open air. Worse at midnight and in the evening and for warmth.	ACONITUM NAPELLUS
With profuse sweating; fainting; body odor.	Persons with nervous nature, yet independent; Better for warmth and fresh air. Worse during day, particularly about 11 a.m.	SULFUR
APPETITE, CRAVING		
Sensation of emptiness, even after a meal.	For salty foods. Better for warmth. Worse at 2 p.m.	CALCAREA CARBONICA
Craving varies with total loss of appetite.	Worse at night.	FERRUM PHOSPHORICUM
Depraved appetite.	For beer.	PULSATILLA NIGRICANS
	Indigestible food, especially in pregnancy.	IGNATIA AMARA
Depraved appetite.	For vinegar.	SEPIA OFFICINALIS

Symptoms/Sensations	Constitutions/Modalities	Remedies
Depraved appetite.	For fats and sugar.	SULFUR
Depraved appetite.	For sour, pungent or high-flavored foods.	HEPAR SULFURIS
Depraved appetite.	Craving at night.	LYCOPODIUM CLAVATUM

APPETITE, LOSS OF

Aversion to all food or craves many indigestible foods, flatulence; hiccough.	Worse in the morning and for smoking. Hunger at night prevents sleep. Moody people.	IGNATIA AMARA
Loss of appetite to all food.	Worse in evening.	RHUS TOXICODENDRON
Bitter taste; tongue coated yellow.	Worse in morning and for cold and beer.	NUX VOMICA
Aversion to meat and warm food; thirst.	Worse in morning. Better for warmth.	SILICA

APPREHENSION

With diarrhea; fear, nervousness; fear of serious disease.	Impulsive people. Prematurely aged look. Worse at menstrual period.	ARGENTUM NITRICUM
With restlessness; anguish; fear of death; hallucinations (sight and smell.)	Worse between midnight and 2 a.m., from cold or food. Better for heat and warm drinks.	ARSENICUM ALBUM
On waking.	Better for cold. Worse in morning and 4 to 5 p.m.	CARBO VEGETABALIS
On making speeches or facing audience.	Persons preferring company. Worse between 4 and 8 p.m.	LYCOPODIUM CLAVATUM
With headache feeling like nail driven in head.	Obsessional persons who can not cut off from problems.	THUJA OCCIDENTALIS
Unable to act—paralyzed by apprehension.	Nervous excitable people. Worse about 10 a.m. Better in open air.	GELSEMIUM SEMPERVIRENS

ARTHRITIS, ACUTE

With much swelling of soft tissues; redness of skin.	Worse for heat and pressure. Better for cold bathing.	APIS MELLIFICA
When arthritic joints are affected by blows or falls.	Worse from least touch, cold, damp and motion. Better for lying down.	ARNICA MONTANA

Symptoms/Sensations	Constitutions/Modalities	Remedies
	Anxious persons who tend to move too fast and have accidents. Worse for warmth and at night. Better from cold pressure.	ARGENTUM NITRICUM
Variable pain.	Worse before midnight. Better from cold	PULSATILLA NIGRICANS
After injections.	Better from cold. Worse at night in warm bed.	LEDUM PALUSTRE

ASTHMA

Spasm prominent all over body, followed by vomiting; giddiness; metallic taste.	Worse before menstruation. Better when perspiring and drinking cold water.	CUPRUM METALLICUM
	Worse in early morning.	NUX VOMICA
Associated with catarrh and cough with little sputum.	Worse about 11 a.m.	IPECACUANHA
With restlessness; fear of suffocation; great exhaustion; fear of being alone.	Attacks occur most intensely between midnight and 2 a.m. Unable to lie down. Worse from cold and after food. Better for warm drinks.	ARSENICUM ALBUM

BACKACHE

From over-exertion or with bruises; rheumatic pain begins low and works up.	Worse for touch, motion and damp cold. Better for lying down or with head low. Bed seems too hard.	ARNICA MONTANA
From uterine infections.		ACTAEA RACEMOSA
Burning pain.	Worse after rest. Better for movement.	CALCAREA FLUORICA
	Worse when sitting and from cold and about 2 p.m.	CALCAREA CARBONICA
With marked stiffness.	Better on movement, for warmth, and firm support. Worse about 7 p.m.	RHUS TOXICODENDRON
Severe, chronic backache.	Better for pressure and cold.	NATRUM MURIATICUM
Low lumbar pains.	Better for warmth. Worse for sitting.	RUTA GRAVEOLENS

Symptoms/Sensations	Constitutions/Modalities	Remedies
Weakness in small of back; drawing in of shoulders.	Worse in wet weather and after midnight. Better for heat and head elevated.	ARSENICUM ALBUM

BALDNESS
(See HAIR LOSS)

BED WETTING
(See INCONTINENCE)

BELCHING

With distended stomach.	Overweight, lazy people. Worse lying down, fatty food, coffee and milk.	CARBO VEGETABALIS
Causing particles of food in mouth with sour, salty taste.	Worse at night and from alcohol. Better lying on right side.	SULFUR
Small belches without relief.	Tired, languid people. Better bending double.	MAGNESIUM PHOSPHORICUM
	With desire for cold drinks. Worse for cold foods.	PHOSPHORUS

BEREAVEMENT

Sudden, unexpected death with shock.	Worse in evening and at night.	ACONITUM NAPELLUS
Prolonged mourning; sighing; sobbing; melancholia.	Worse in the morning. Quiet, brooding people inclined to be uncommunicative.	IGNATIA AMARA

BILIOUS ATTACK

With constipation, frontal headache, depression, and sharp pains in liver. Food lies like a stone in stomach.	Dark haired persons. Worse about 3 a.m. Better for lying down.	BRYONIA ALBA
With constipation and depression after over-eating or drinking.	Dark, sallow, irritable sedentary persons. Better in the evening.	NUX VOMICA
Sharp pains in liver; pains in loins; constipation.	Worse before breakfast and from motion.	BERBERIS VULGARIS
Stools in minute lumps with discomfort in region of liver.	Better for hot water and temporary relief when eating. Worse very early morning.	CHELIDONIUM MAJUS

Symptoms/Sensations	Constitutions/Modalities	Remedies
BITES		
From animals; anxiety; fear.	Immediately, take	ACONITUM NAPELLUS
Tarantula bite.	Better for warm applications.	LACHESIS MUTUS
Mosquito and spider bites.		APIS MELLIFICA
With injured nerves; puncture wound.	Worse from touch.	HYPERICUM PERFORATUM
(See also STINGS)		
BLADDER DISORDERS		
Burning pains.		CANTHARIS VESTICATORIA
Burning, cutting pains in urethra; during or after urination; frequent desire to pass water.	Especially women. Dislike of darkness.	BERBERIS VULGARIS
BLISTERS		
Blistering burns and scalds.	Worse from touch or approach.	CANTHARIS VESICATORIA
With burning sensations; itching; swelling.	Better for warmth. Worse for cold.	ARSENICUM ALBUM
With purple or blue tinge; dark blisters.	Especially left side.	LACHESIS MUTUS
Blisters (vesicles) on lips; fever blisters.	Worse about 10 a.m., and from heat. Better in open air.	NATRUM MURIATICUM
BODY ODOR		
Sour, sticky sweat; skin sensitive to touch; sweats day and night.	Persons with fair hair and complexion. Worse about 5 to 6 p.m.	HEPAR SULFURIS
With itching; eczema. Sweats easily.	Nervous, yet independent persons. Worse about 11 a.m. and from heat.	SULFUR
(See also PERSPIRATION)		
BOILS		
Boils in sensitive areas. Bruised sensation; itching, burning eruptions.	Worse from touch. Worse from cold.	ANRICA MONTANA
Boils are slow developing. Promotes expulsion of pus.	Persons who feel chilly. Better for warmth.	SILICA
Redness and swelling around boils; burning, stinging sensation.	Worse for heat in any form and pressure. Better in open air.	APIS MELLIFICA

Symptoms/Sensations	Constitutions/Modalities	Remedies
With burning sensations; malignant; itching.	Worse from cold or scratching. Better for heat.	ARSENICUM ALBUM
Boils on back.		PHYTOLACCA DECANDRA
Very painful, with blue tinge.	Worse after sleep. Better for warm applications.	LACHESIS MUTUS
When skin injuries turn septic. Blisters turn into boils. Boils are hot.	Fair persons who feel chilly. Worse for cold. Better for warmth.	HEPAR SULFURIS

BONE PAINS

Pains in small areas, especially bones of the head.	Better for heat; worse in morning.	KALI BICHROMICUM
Pains of the mandible.	Worse during evening.	PHOSPHORUS
Recovery from bone injuries and sprains.	Better for warmth.	RUTA GRAVEOLENS
Spinal pains.	Slim, week children. Worse for cold.	SILICA

BREATH, BAD

Fetid breath; bitter taste.	Worse for wine and at rest.	ARNICA MONTANA
With metallic taste.	Worse at night.	MERCURIUS VIVUS
Bad odor after dinner.	Dark, slim persons; inclined to be impatient. Worse for beer.	NUX VOMICA
Sour smelling breath; fetid; with bitter taste on waking.	Worse from physical exertion and early morning. Better for rest.	KALI PHOSPHORICUM
With thick, yellow-coated tongue; liverish.	Worse in early morning. Better after meals.	CHELIDONIUM MAJUS

BREATHING DIFFICULTY

With dry throat and chesty cold; burning throat.	Better when sitting or bending forward or head elevated. Worse from cold, wet weather and after midnight.	ARSENICUM ALBUM
	Worse for heat. Robust people.	LEDUM PALUSTRE

(See also ASTHMA)

BRONCHITIS

With hoarseness or loss of voice; wheezing.	Tall, slim persons with pale, delicate skin; worse for talking.	PHOSPHORUS

Symptoms/Sensations	Constitutions/Modalities	Remedies
In early stages, dry, tickling cough; irritation in throat on exposure to cold; restlessness.	Better in open air. Worse in dry, cold winds and in the evening and at night.	ACONITUM NAPELLUS
Dry, hacking cough; pains between shoulders; sharp chest pains; constipation; headache.	Dark-haired persons with dark complexion. May be rheumatic. Worse after meals. Better for cold.	BRYONIA ALBA
Redness and hot face; high temperature.	Lively, congenial persons; worse at night.	ATROPA BELLADONNA
Loose cough; tendency to perspiration; red, sore, burning throat.	Worse at night, after drinking and in wet, damp weather.	MERCURIUS VIVUS
Spasmodic cough; persistent nausea; rattling of mucus in bronchial tubes.	Worse at night and about 11 a.m.	IPECACUANHA
Acute or chronic bronchitis where mucus is tough and stringy.	Worse in morning or in hot weather.	KALI BICHROMICUM
Profuse expectoration.	Worse on lying down or in warm room. Delicate, blond persons.	PULSATILLA NIGRICANS
Later stages of bronchitis. Profuse expectoration.	Worse in bed at night. Older persons with cold extremities.	SULFUR CARBO VEGETABILIS

BRUISES

Symptoms/Sensations	Constitutions/Modalities	Remedies
All types of bruises, particularly of soft parts; skin black and blue.	Use Arnica ointment externally. Worse for least touch.	*ARNICA MONTANA*
Bruised bones and tendons.	Worse from cold.	RUTA GRAVEOLENS
Bruises on fingers and toes.	Worse from cold and touch.	HYPERICUM PERFORATUM
With broken skin over bruise.	Worse in warm air.	HAMAMELIS VIRGINIANA
From blow with blunt instrument causing bruise without penetration of skin. Blows on eye.		SYMPHYTUM OFFICINALIS

BUNIONS

Symptoms/Sensations	Constitutions/Modalities	Remedies
Hard, true bunions caused by pressure.	Persons with fine skin; light complexion. Worse for cold.	SILICA
With gout.	Worse on beginning to move. Better for warmth.	RHUS TOXICODENDRON

Symptoms/Sensations	Constitutions/Modalities	Remedies
BURNS		
All types of burns, before blisters form.	Worse from touch and after drinking cold water.	CANTHARIS VESICATORIA
Infected burns; cannot bear to be uncovered.	Sensitive persons with fair hair and complexion. Better for warmth. Worse about 5 to 6 p.m.	HEPAR SULFURIS
Superficial burns, scalds.	Pain relief, healing.	URTICA URENS
BURSITIS		
Acute bursitis		APIS MELLIFICA
Chronic bursitis	Locally, Rhus Tox. ointment.	RHUS TOXICODENDRON
CANDIDA INFECTION		
Eruptions in patches or single infected areas of raised red spots.	Particularly babies or breast-feeding mothers.	Dry skin and expose to air and light. Keep skin cool. CALENDULA OFFICINALIS ointment or cream.
As above. Diaper rash.	Baby is irritable, fractious, tearful.	CHAMOMILLA
Bright red patches; swelling; feverish.	Worse for touch or motion; worse on right side; worse at 3 pm and 10 pm to midnight. Better for lying down.	ATROPA BELLADONNA
Mouth inflamed; soreness; spongy gums; coated tongue; restless; metallic taste.	Worse for heat. People who tire easily. Better for cold drink.	MERCURIUS VIVUS
Mouth inflamed; burning sensation; soreness.	Worse for eating and about 11 a.m. Independent people who perspire easily with body odor.	SULFUR
CAPRICIOUSNESS		
	Dark-haired persons with dark complexion. Worse in heat.	BRYONIA ALBA
	Particularly children and teething infants.	CHAMOMILLA
During pregnancy.	Worse in the morning.	IPECACUANHA

Symptoms/Sensations	Constitutions/Modalities	Remedies

CARBUNCLES

With shiny redness and throbbing or stabbing pains.	Worse about 3 p.m.	ATROPA BELLADONNA
With blueness or purple surroundings.	Worse after sleep and for pressure.	LACHESIS MUTUS
When discharge commences; intense pain; burning; green underlying tissue.	Worse for warmth.	SILICA
With thickening.	Worse from touch and cold air. Better for warmth.	HEPAR SULFURIS
Dark blue, black appearance of carbuncle; bruised sensation.	Worse from least touch and motion.	ARNICA MONTANA

CATARRH

Yellow, stringy catarrh; sore throat; hoarseness.	Worse in the morning between 4 and 5 a.m.	KALI BICHROMICUM
Thick, yellow-green catarrah; head cold.	Worse after rest and from cold.	CALCAREA FLUORICA
With watering eyes and runny nose.	Worse in the evening and in bed.	EUPHRASIA OFFICINALIS
With unhealthy complexion and constipation.	Chilly persons. Worse lying down and about 10 to 11 a.m.	NATRUM MURIATICUM
With skin eruptions around nostrils; constipation.	Cautious persons. Worse at night.	GRAPHITES
Variable intensity; discharge clear or yellow.	Worse in the evening and at night. Better for cool room.	PULSATILLA NIGRICANS

CHAPPED SKIN

	Use Calendula cream externally.	CALENDULA OFFICINALIS

CHEST CONGESTION

With hoarseness and loss of voice.	Tall, slim, perhaps young persons. Worse during afternoon.	PHOSPHORUS
With dry, painful cough.	Worse for any warmth, motion or exertion. Better for rest.	BRYONIA ALBA
With rheumatic pains; depression.		ACTAEA RACEMOSA

Symptoms/Sensations	*Constitutions/Modalities*	*Remedies*
CHICKEN POX		
	Weepy persons with little thirst. Worse about 4 p.m.	PULSATILLA NIGRICANS
At onset of symptoms; blistering, itching; restlessness.	Worse after midnight. Better for warmth.	RHUS TOXICODENDRON
CHILBLAINS		
Bright red chilblains; swelling.	Worse about 10 p.m. to midnight or during afternoon.	ATROPA BELLADONNA
Simple chilblains with itching and burning.	Especially girls with delayed menses. Worse in evening.	PULSATILLA NIGRICANS
Inflamed; red, with much itching and burning; blistering; tingling in feet.	Worse in cold, wet weather, at night and lying on back. Better for motion, warm applications and stretching out foot. Use TAMUS ointment externally.	RHUS TOXICODENDRON
CHILLS (see COLDS)		
COCCYX PAIN		
As a result of a fall; pain radiating up spine.	Better bending head backward. Worse in cold or from touch.	HYPERICUM PERFORATUM
Burning, stinging pain.	Worse for touch or pressure. Better for cold bathing or about 4 to 6 p.m.	APIS MELLIFICA
Pain in coccyx and sacrum, extending up and down.	Worse when sitting, walking or with touch.	KALI BICHROMICUM
Weak spine, susceptible to drafts.	Worse on lying down and cold. Better for warmth.	SILICA
COLDS		
Sudden onset of cold; in early stages, after exposure to cold; after chill feeling has passed; sneezing; thirsty for large amounts of water. Alternating coldness and heat.	Worse in cold, dry winds and in evening and midnight. Better for rest.	ACONITUM NAPELLUS

Symptoms/Sensations	Constitutions/Modalities	Remedies
Sneezing and runny nose.	Worse in evening and after midnight.	EUPHRASIA OFFICINALIS
Sneezing; nose runs like tap. Influenza-like cold.	Worse in morning. Persons with pale, oily skin.	NATRUM MURIATICUM
Well developed cold with thick discharge; after exposure to cold and damp; much sneezing.	Worse at night and in wet weather.	MERCURIUS VIVUS
Thin, irritating discharge; sore nostrils; lassitude; nose feels stopped up.	Worse between 1 and 2 p.m., from cold, wet weather. Better for warmth and warm drinks.	ARSENICUM ALBUM
With loss of smell.	Better for warmth. Worse around 11 a.m.	SULFUR
With inflamed, swollen, painful nose; thick, yellow catarrh; hoarseness; in later stages of colds.	Worse for slightest draft. Better for wrapping up head and warmth.	HEPAR SULFURIS
With intermittent catarrh.	Better outdoors. Blue-eyed, fair-haired persons.	PULSATILLA NIGRICANS
Hard, dry cough; stitching pain in chest; thirsty.	Worse for cold and about 3 a.m.	BRYONIA ALBA
Chest congested; early stages of colds with no definite symptoms.	Better for gentle exercise. Worse at night, especially 4 to 6 a.m.	FERRUM PHOSPHORICUM
Influenza-like cold; aching; trembling. Chills up and down spine.	Worse in morning. Better outdoors.	GELSEMIUM SEMPERVIRENS

COLITIS

With watery stools.	Worse by sight or smell or food; motion and loss of sleep. Better for stooping.	COLCHICUM AUTUMNALE
	Worse after midnight and between 1 and 2 p.m. Better for warmth and warm drinks.	ARSENICUM ALBUM
Feeling of stool remaining in rectum.	Intolerant persons. Better for sleep. Worse for coffee.	NUX VOMICA
Burning pain; nausea; vomiting.	Worse for touch.	CANTHARIS VESICATORIA
Where abdomen is distended; hot; painful	Worse from touch and when lying down. Better when semi-erect.	ATROPA BELLADONNA

Symptoms/Sensations	Constitutions/Modalities	Remedies
COLLAPSE		
Head hot; sweating; car exhaust poisioning. Moisten lips with liquid.	Better for air.	CARBO VEGETABILIS
COMMON COLD (see COLDS)		
CONCUSSION		
First aid treatment; with visible bruising; delirious state; objects whirl about.	Worse from touch or motion. Better lying down or with head held low.	ARNICA MONTANA
With persistent insomnia.	Better for warmth.	KALI PHOSPHORICUM
If head is very heavy and sensitive; with painful wounds.	Worse for any touch or movement and cold.	HYPERICUM PERFORATUM
Flushed, red face; high temperature; restlessness.	Better in open air.	ACONITUM NAPELLUS (May follow Arnica.)
CONJUNCTIVITIS		(Frequent bathing with hot water is advantageous.)
Acute inflammation of eyes from cold or injury. Eyes dry and hot as if sand in them.	Worse for light. Worse for cold, dry winds. Worse from tobacco smoke.	ACONTIUM NAPELLUS
If no improvement after 48 hours, cannot bear bright light.	Worse in evening.	EUPHRASIA OFFICINALIS
With headaches; spots before eyes; swelling; eye strain; acute granular conjunctivitis.	Desire for sweets. Worse for warmth and at night. Better for fresh air.	ARGENTUM NITRICUM
Inflamed eyes through weeping and rubbing of eyes.	Fair, blue-eyed, sensitive persons.	PULSATILLA NIGRICANS
Associated with shingles.	Worse about 7 p.m.	RHUS TOXICODENDRON
Eye red, bloodshot; dilated pupils.	Worse at night, particularly before midnight.	GRAPHITES
CONSTIPATION		(Diet and exercise are recommended.)

Symptoms/Sensations	Constitutions/Modalities	Remedies
With large, hard, dry stools; painful; during pregnancy.	With thirst. Worse for bread.	BRYONIA ALBA
With ineffectual urging; black, hard stools.	Dark, sedentary persons; pregnant women. Worse from cold foods.	NUX VOMICA
Stool recedes when partly expelled; light color; nausea.	Pale, slim children. Worse from alcohol.	SILICA
Large, hard, knotty stool; delayed menses; discharge of mucus and blood.	Worse at night.	GRAPHITES
With distention of abdomen; flatulence; very hard, small, difficult stools; rumblings in bowels; ringing in ears.	Conscientious persons; persons with pale complexion and slim face. Worse between 4 and 6 p.m.	LYCOPODIUM CLAVATUM
Debility; headache, hard lumpy stools; long-lasting pain in rectum; fainting.	Sedentary persons after an active life.	HYDRASTIS CANADENSIS

COUGH

Symptoms/Sensations	Constitutions/Modalities	Remedies
Short, dry, irritating cough.	Better in open air. Worse at night, from tobacco smoke and dry, cold winds.	ACONITUM NAPELLUS
Dry cough with pain in chest.	Worse on laying down at night; on entering warm room.	BRYONIA ALBA
Sudden attacks; whooping cough; with laryngitis; vomiting; spasmodic cough.	Worse when lying down, with warmth, or midnight to 3 a.m.	DROSERA ROTUNDIFOLIA
Dry cough; hoarseness; loss of voice; worse when talking.	Worse for getting wet, in the evening, lying on left side. Better lying on right side.	PHOSPHORUS
Choking cough; nausea; vomiting.	Worse about 11 a.m.	IPECACUANHA
With stringy sputum; metallic, hacking cough.	Better from heat. Worse in morning.	KALI BICHROMICUM
Irritating cough with redness of face; feeling of soreness in larynx.	Worse in evening and early night on lying down.	ATROPA BELLADONNA

Symptoms/Sensations	Constitutions/Modalities	Remedies
CRAMP		
From fatigue; in the calves; in the muscles. In soles.	Worse for touch and damp cold. Worse for motion and loss of sleep. Better for stooping.	ARNICA MONTANA COLCHICUM AUTUMNALE
Beginning as twitches; especially in fingers and toes; cramp extending into chest during period; cramp in palms.	Better when perspiring. Worse before and during periods.	*CUPRUM METALLICUM*
Stomach cramp; loss of appetite; nausea; constipation.	Better for a short nap. Worse for pressure.	NUX VOMICA
CROUP		
In early stages; restlessness; anxiety.	Worse in dry, cold air and in evening and at night. Better in open air.	ACONITUM NAPELLUS
Rattling, choking cough.	Worse after midnight. Worse for cold air or slightest draft. Better for wrapping up head and warmth.	HEPAR SULFURIS
Croupy cough; red face and dry mouth.	Worse about 3 p.m. Lively, red-faced people.	ATROPA BELLADONNA
Brought on by fright or emotion; dry spasmodic cough.	Worse in the morning, after meals and for external warmth. Better while eating.	IGNATIA AMARA
With tough, stringy, yellowish expectoration; difficult to bring up.	Worse about 2 to 3 a.m.	KALI BICHROMICUM
CUTS (See WOUNDS)		
CYSTITIS		
Irritable bladder; with desire to urinate; slight burning sensation and soreness when urinating.	Worse from 4 to 6 p.m. and after sleeping.	APIS MELLIFICA
Constant desire to urinate, even a few drops; inflammation; urine scalds; smarting, burning sensation.	Worse for drinking cold water or coffee.	*CANTHARIS VESICATORIA*

Symptoms/Sensations	Constitutions/Modalities	Remedies
DANDRUFF		
Dry dandruff; white.	Persons who perspire easily; face oily and shiny.	THUJA OCCIDENTALIS
Moist dandruff.	Worse during day.	SEPIA OFFICINALIS
Itching dandruff.	Persons with thick hair; worse at night.	SULFUR
Very scaly with moistness and crusting; sensation of cobwebs on head.	Worse after menstruation.	GRAPHITES
Itching, scaly dandruff.	Worse for heat. Better for rubbing.	CANTHARIS VESICATORIA
DEAFNESS		
With discharge from ears; eczema on outer ear.	Worse between 4 and 8 p.m. Better for warmth.	LYCOPODIUM CLAVATUM
Catarrhal deafness.	Better in open air. Worse about 4 p.m.	PULSATILLA NIGRICANS
Catarrhal deafness with sinusitis.	Slim children. Better for warmth.	SILICA
Slow to improve; roaring in ears.	Elderly, easily tired people.	HYDRASTIS CANADENSIS
With roaring noises in ear.	Worse in noisy environment.	GRAPHITES
DEBILITY		
After acute disease; exhaustion.	Slim children with dark hair. Touchy persons who tend to be absentminded.	CALCAREA PHOSPHORICA
With flushing to head and face; mental exhaustion.	Pale, delicate persons who prefer to be alone.	FERRUM PHOSPHORICUM
	Fat, pale children.	CALCAREA CARBONICA
	Slim, rickety children.	SILICA
DEPRESSION		
From bereavement or worry; change of life; full of contradictions.	Emotional persons, who tend to be moody and uncommunicative. Worse in the morning.	IGNATIA AMARA
Despondency; as if black pall over everything; confusion.	Better when eating.	ACTAEA RACEMOSA

Symptoms/Sensations	Constitutions/Modalities	Remedies
Depression during menses or after food; emotional state.	Worse on lying down at night; wants to be alone.	NATRUM MURIATICUM
Acute melancholia.	Normally lively and congenial persons. Worse at 3 p.m. and at night.	ATROPA BELLADONNA
Dyspeptic; melancholia.	Worse between 4 and 8 p.m.; persons who prefer company.	LYCOPODIUM CLAVATUM
Associated with bad temper.	Persons inclined to be impatient. Better in evening. Worse before 3 a.m.	NUX VOMICA
Depressed and irritable; overcome by responsibilities.	Especially women. Worse during daytime.	SEPIA OFFICINALIS
DIARRHEA		(Note: Proper diet is always recommended.)
White, slimy diarrhea; stomach ache.	Persons who are easily angered.	CHAMOMILLA
Acute diarrhea with nausea; vomiting at smell, thought, or sight of food, especially fish; coldness in stomach.	Worse for motion, sundown to sunrise.	COLCHICUM AUTUMNALE
Diarrhea in morning; yellow with smell of bad eggs.	Worse in early morning, particularly around 11 a.m.	SULFUR
From mild food poisoning; simultaneous diarrhea and vomiting; dark, bloody diarrhea.	Worse from food, cold drinks and after midnight. Better for heat and warm drinks.	ARSENICUM ALBUM
Greenish-yellow diarrhea.	Worse in morning.	APIS MELLIFICA
From artificial food; vomiting.	Especially in infants.	NUX VOMICA
Caused by fear; flatulence; belching; nausea.	Worse after eating, particularly sweet foods and during menstrual period. Desire for candies.	ARGENTUM NITRICUM

DISTENDED ABDOMEN
(see ABDOMEN, DISTENDED)

DRY MOUTH

| With thirst. | Worse about 3 a.m. | BRYONIA ALBA |

Symptoms/Sensations	Constitutions/Modalities	Remedies
Without thirst; tongue red and swollen; swollen lips (especially upper).	Worse from 4 to 6 p.m. and after sleeping. Better for cold.	APIS MELLIFICA

DYSPEPSIA

From indigestible food; flatulence; vomiting; constipation; hangover.	Dark-complected, irritable persons. Better in evening. Worse after food and alcohol.	NUX VOMICA
With flatulence; cutting pains; acidity; tendency to diarrhea.	Chilly persons who like open air. Worse from butter.	CARBO VEGETABILIS
Sensation of stone in stomach; pain between shoulders or across the forehead; constipation.	Dark-haired persons with tendency to rheumatism; worse about 3 a.m. and 9 p.m.	BRYONIA ALBA
Bilious dyspepsia with irritability.	Worse around 9 a.m.	CHAMOMILLA
With thick, yellow tongue; red underside; beer drinkers.	Worse in morning and from alcohol.	KALI BICHROMICUM
From nervous excitement; with flatulence; belching, radiating pains.	Worse from cold food, sweets and at night and during menstruation.	ARGENTUM NITRICUM
Stomach burning; great thirst—drinking much in small quantities; stomach feels 'raw'; fear.	Better for hot drinks. Craving for milk, acid substances and coffee. Worse from alcohol.	ARSENICUM ALBUM

EARACHE

From cold winds, with inflammation; sensitive to noises. Sensations of water in left ear.	Worse in evening and at night and lying on affected ear.	ACONITUM NAPELLUS
With redness, heat and throbbing.	Worse about 3 p.m. Better for warmth.	ATROPA BELLADONNA
Pain intolerable.	Worse for warmth and at night.	CHAMOMILLA
With sore throat; ear wax hard.	Worse when swallowing and after sleep. Better for warm applications.	LACHESIS MUTUS

EAR INFLAMMATION
(See OTITIS)

ECZEMA

Palms of hands; behind ears; cracked skin	Cautious people. Worse at night.	GRAPHITES

Symptoms/Sensations	Constitutions/Modalities	Remedies
Dry eczema.	Worse for scratching. Better for heat.	ARSENICUM ALBUM
Weeping eczema.	Scrofulous children. Worse at night and wet weather.	MERCURIUS VIVUS
Chronic eczema; very sensitive to touch.	Worse for cold. Better for warmth.	HEPAR SULFURIS
With vesicles	Worse after midnight.	RHUS TOXICODENDRON
Dry eczema; itching; scratching; causes burning.	Worse in bed at night. Better for cold air. Worse on left side.	SULFUR
At borders of hair.	People with pale, oily skin. Better in open air. Worse mid-morning.	NATRUM MURIATICUM

EMOTIONAL PROBLEMS

Capriciousness; rapidly changing moods; worry and its effects; grief or disappointment.	Worse in the morning and from coffee. Emotional, sensitive persons who prefer to be alone. Better for eating.	IGNATIA AMARA
Worry about coming events; trembling; nervousness; melancholia; poor memory.	Impulsive, nervous persons. Desire for sweets. Cannot tolerate heat.	ARGENTUM NITRICUM
Gloom; despondency; tendency to suicide; cannot concentrate.		ACTAEA RACEMOSA
Sinking feeling in stomach; dejected; loss of memory; fretful; irritable.	Before noon, particularly 11 a.m.; worse for warmth.	SULFUR

(see also ANGER, APPREHENSION, BEREAVEMENT, DEPRESSION, FEAR, HYSTERIA, MENOPAUSE)

ENTERITIS

(see DIARRHEA)

EXCITEMENT

With fever and restlessness.	Better in open air. Worse for music and in evening and at night.	ACONITUM NAPELLUS

Symptoms/Sensations	Constitutions/Modalities	Remedies
With throbbing headache.	Lively persons. Worse from noise and about 3 p.m.	ATROPA BELLADONNA
Easily excited, with tears.	Fair haired females; affectionate persons; children.	PULSATILLA NIGRICANS
Causing loss of sleep.	Particularly children.	CHAMOMILLA

EXHAUSTION, MENTAL

From excessive mental effort.	Better for warmth.	KALI PHOSPHORICUM
With headache; loss of memory from overwork; dread of mental effort.	Worse from cold; better for warmth.	SILICA
After considerable worry or sickness.	Pale persons. Worse from cold.	CALCAREA PHOSPHORICUM
Dull, sluggish feeling.	Excitable, nervous people. Worse in morning, particularly 10 to 11 a.m.	GELSEMIUM SEMPERVIRENS

EXHAUSTION, PHYSICAL

From overexertion or after diarrhea or sickness; angina pectoris.	Worse for motion, touch and cold. Better lying down with head low.	ARNICA MONTANA

EYE INFLAMMATION
(See CONJUNCTIVITIS)

EYE INJURY

Traumatic injuries or blows to the eyes with blunt instrument.	Immediately, take	*SYMPHYTUM OFFICINALIS*

FAINTING

Hysterical fainting; from worry.	Emotional, sensitive persons; easily moved to tears; worse in the morning.	IGNATIA AMARA
Due to debility; restlessness; sweating; anguish; lacking courage to perform task.	Worse in cold, wet weather or from food. Better with head elevated and warm drinks.	ARSENICUM ALBUM
Due to fright, fear; emotional excitement.	Better in open air. Worse in warm room.	ACONITUM NAPELLUS

FAT EXCESS
(See OBESITY)

Symptoms/Sensations	Constitutions/Modalities	Remedies
FEAR		
Fear of death; sudden fright; congestion of the head.	Worse in evening and on waking at night. Better in open air.	ACONITUM NAPELLUS
Fear causing diarrhea; examination panic; stage fright; nervousness; fear of serious disease.	Irritable, nervous persons, prematurely aged look. Worse at night and during menstrual period.	ARGENTUM NITRICUM
Anguish with cries and tears; nightmares.	Worse at night, particularly 3 a.m.	ATROPA BELLADONNA
From fright; stomach upset; headache; convulsions (especially children).	Emotional, sensitive persons.	IGNATIA AMARA
Great fear to point of terror; fear to death; fear of being left alone; cold sweat.	Precise persons. Worse between 1 and 2 a.m. and for disorder or confusion. Better for warmth.	ARSENICUM ALBUM
Fear of coming event; worry about coping with life and school.	Nervous people. Worse in morning, particularly about 10 a.m.	GELSEMIUM SEMPERVIRENS
FEET, DISCOMFORT		
Aching from walking long distance; gout; soreness from walking.	Worse from rest or motion and cold.	ARNICA MONTANA
Burning in the soles.	Worse when walking.	GRAPHITES
Hot feet with burning sensation.	Worse in the evening in bed; better for cold air.	SULFUR
Cramps in the feet; tearing in instep and big toe; gout; coldness of feet.	Worse at night and for motion.	COLCHICUM AUTUMNALE
Tearing in the heels; excessive perspiration and smelly; soreness of soles.		SILICA
Profuse perspiration causing soreness.	Weakened; depressive; slim-faced persons with pale complexion.	LYCOPODIUM CLAVATUM
Swollen feet with stinging sensations; stiffness. Feet feel too large.	Better for cold bathing. Worse for heat and pressure.	APIS MELLIFICA
Hot and sweating.		CHAMOMILLA

FINGERS
(See WHITLOWS)

Symptoms/Sensations	Constitutions/Modalities	Remedies

FLATULENCE

Coming up from stomach causing difficulty in breathing or pains about chest.	Overweight people. Worse in evening. Better for cold.	CARBO VEGETABILIS
In lower part of body; constipation.	Worse for cold food.	LYCOPODIUM CLAVATUM
Wind easily coming away through mouth; from eating fats and salty foods; eating too fast; diarrhea.	Worse for heat and after eating cold foods. Better for cold, fresh air. Impulsive people.	ARGENTUM NITRICUM
After bringing up wind. (See also ABDOMEN, DISTENDED, and DYSPEPSIA)	Irritable children.	CHAMOMILLA

FRACTURES

When bones are bruised; dislocations.	Worse lying down and in cold air.	RUTA GRAVEOLENS
To assist the union of fractures; irritability of bone at fracture; injuries to sinews and tendons.		SYMPHYTUM OFFICINALIS
When fracture is slow to heal.	Scrofulous subjects.	CALCAREA PHOSPHORICA

GENITAL CONDITIONS
(see SEXUAL PROBLEMS)

GIDDINESS

Tendency to pitch forward; biliousness.	Worse from any movement, warmth, and at about 3 a.m.	BRYONIA ALBA
From rush of blood to the head; effects of sun.	Worse at night. Better for cold applications and slow movement.	FERRUM PHOSPHORICUM
On looking up or going up stairs.	Worse for physical or mental exertion and on standing.	CALCAREA CARBONICA
From exhaustion.	Worse after mental effort. Better for warmth.	KALI PHOSPHORICUM
On arising in morning.	Better for warmth and sitting erect.	ATROPA BELLADONNA

GINGIVITIS

Swollen, tender gums; bleed easily.		CALCAREA PHOSPHORICA

Symptoms/Sensations	Constitutions/Modalities	Remedies
With great thirst; gums bleed easily; metallic taste; dry tongue.	Worse after midnight to 2 p.m. Better for warmth.	ARSENICUM ALBUM
Swollen gums; bad breath; inflammation; sweet, metallic taste.	Worse at night.	MERCURIUS VIVUS
With mouth ulcers.	Better for wrapping up head and after eating.	HEPAR SULFURIS

GOUT

Enlargements of joints of fingers.	Worse from cold.	CALCAREA FLUORICA
Most cases of gout; usually swelling of the big toe; dejection; weakness; nausea; swelling.	Worse by movement and at night.	COLCHICUM AUTUMNALE
In the early stages; foot red, inflamed, swollen.	Worse from heat, fatty foods, allowing foot to hang down and about 4 p.m. Better for cold applications.	PULSATILLA NIGRICANS
Acute gout; intense burning and itching; swelling.	Worse for touch and cold.	URTICA URENS
Pain shoots through foot. Ball of big toe swollen.	Better from cold air and putting feet in cold water. Worse at night.	LEDUM PALUSTRE

GRIEF
(see BEREAVEMENT)

GRINDING OF TEETH

With hot, dry skin; feverish.	Worse in afternoon and on lying down.	ATROPA BELLADONNA

HAIR LOSS

Baldness; sudden onset; anxiety; sensation of cold spot on forehead.	Take internally and apply externally.	ARNICA MONTANA
With very greasy hair.		BRYONIA ALBA
General baldness.	Dark-haired persons. Take internally and apply externally to affected part.	SEPIA OFFICINALIS

HALITOSIS
(See BREATH, BAD)

HANGOVER
(see ALCOHOLISM)

Symptoms/Sensations	Constitutions/Modalities	Remedies
HAY FEVER		
With fever and prostration and as prophylactic.	Worse in open air and cold. Better indoors, from heat and warm drinks.	ARSENICUM ALBUM
With burning lachrymations.	Worse in the evening and in bright light.	EUPHRASIA OFFICINALIS
With nasal obstruction.	Worse on waking; chilly persons. Better for warmth.	SILICA
With red, stinging, swollen eyelids.	Better for cold bathing. Worse for heat and in late afternoon between 4 and 6 p.m.	APIS MELLIFICA
HEADACHE		
With dizziness; feeling of big head; coldness; trembling; from mental exertion or dancing.	Impulsive, nervous people. Better for pressure, cold and fresh air. Worse for warmth and at night.	ARGENTUM NITRICUM
In forehead; throbbing headache; heavy eyelids; flushed face; sense of burning in eyeballs.	Worse by light, noise and movement around 3 p.m. Better when sitting.	ATROPA BELLADONNA
Painful, watering eyes; cannot bear bright lights.	Better in open air. Worse in evening, indoors and bright light.	EUPHRASIA OFFICINALIS
Headache over one eye, especially right eye; blurred sight.	Better for warmth. Worse about 2 to 3 a.m.	KALI BICHROMICUM
Over left eye; acidity.	Better for cold. Worse about 4 to 5 p.m.	CARBO VEGETABILIS
Heavy-pressure headache; giddiness; constipation; tension in the neck.	Worse for mental exhaustion, drinking alcohol, eating or on waking. Better for sleep.	NUX VOMICA
Headache from loss of sleep, worry, or mental strain; in eyeballs.	Better in open air.	ACTAEA RACEMOSA
Pressure headache on right side over right eye.	Better in evening after 8 p.m.	CHELIDONIUM MAJUS followed by LYCOPODIUM CLAVATUM
Throbbing headache; variable; indigestion of starchy and fatty food.	Better for cold, open air, and walking. Worse for looking up.	PULSATILLA NIGRICANS

Symptoms/Sensations	Constitutions/Modalities	Remedies
	School children. Worse about 2 p.m.	CALCAREA PHOSPHORICA
Chronic headache; sensitive to pressure; loss of memory from overwork; sometimes sore eyeballs; sweating.	Worse for noise, movement, and light. Better for warmth.	SILICA
	Worse for any movement and about 3 a.m.	BRYONIA ALBA

HEMORRHOIDS

Bleeding piles with loose bowels; soreness.	Worse during day and in warm, moist air.	HAMAMELIS VIRGINIANA
With blood and mucus.	Worse at night and in wet, damp weather.	MERCURIUS VIVUS
Burning; itching; warts; swollen hemorrhoids.	Worse from cold and at 3 a.m. and 3 p.m. Worse for sitting and walking.	THUJA OCCIDENTALIS
Itching piles; large; burning; stinging; constipation.	Irritable persons; worse between midnight and 2 a.m.	NUX VOMICA
Itching; burning, particularly after hard stool; covered in blood.	Women with tendency to rheumatism. Worse for standing.	BERBERIS VULGARIS

HERPES

Eruptions about lips.	Worse about 10 a.m. and by seashore.	NATRUM MURIATICUM
Herpes zoster (shingles) on back or side or on head.	Especially middle-aged persons.	RHUS TOXICODENDRON
Scurfy herpes; in isolated spots.	Particularly women. Worse for washing and sweating.	SEPIA OFFICINALIS
Chronic herpes zoster; anguish; restlessness; exhaustion.	Worse from cold, after midnight. Better for heat.	ARSENICUM ALBUM

HICCOUGH

Ordinary acute cases; occurring an hour or two after food.	Worse after meals.	NUX VOMICA
Chronic cases; with multiple spasms or neuralgic pains; thirst for cold drinks.	Worse from cold and at night. Better from bending double and warmth.	MAGNESIA PHOSPHORICUM

Symptoms/Sensations	Constitutions/Modalities	Remedies
Hiccough after eating, drinking, or smoking; hysteria.	Worse in morning.	IGNATIA AMARA
With chronic dyspepsia.	Worse between 4 and 8 p.m. Slim-faced persons.	LYCOPODIUM CLAVATUM

HOARSENESS

From overexertion and overuse of voice; raw, sore feeling in throat; after shock.	Prefers to be alone.	ARNICA MONTANA
Following overexcitement or hysteria.	Worse in the morning and in open air.	IGNATIA AMARA
From overuse of voice.	Better for warmth.	KALI PHOSPHORICUM
With laryngitis.		PHOSPHORUS
From a cold; in early stages of hoarseness; swollen, dry tonsils.	Better in open air. Worse in warm room and in dry, cold winds.	ACONITUM NAPELLUS

HYPOCHONDRIA

With depression; suicidal tendency; black cloud over everything; despondency.	Worse in cold. Better in warmth.	ACTAEA RACEMOSA
With tendency to hysteria.	Emotional, sensitive persons.	IGNATIA AMARA
Melancholic; tired of life.	Prefers to be alone. Worse when lying down.	NATRUM MURIATICUM
Quarrelsome; inclined to violence; dry skin; craving for sweet foods; digestive problems.	Intelligent, sedentary persons.	LYCOPODIUM CLAVATUM

HYSTERIA

From worry; grief; lump in throat; capriciousness.	Impressionable persons who tend to be moody and cannot communicate.	IGNATIA AMARA
Craving sensations; depressed; suicidal tendency.		ACTAEA RACEMOSA
Very talkative; delirium tremens; confusion.	People with melancholic disposition. Worse for tight clothing and after sleep.	LACHESIS MUTUS

IMPOTENCE
(See SEXUAL PROBLEMS)

Symptoms/Sensations	Constitutions/Modalities	Remedies
INCONTINENCE		
Simple incontinence during deep sleep.	Worse 10 p.m. to midnight	ATROPA BELLADONNA
Shortly after going to sleep.	Dark-haired persons, especially women. Better for warmth.	SEPIA OFFICINALIS
Dribbling while sitting, walking, or coughing, and at night.	Fair-haired, blue-eyed women, tending to overweight.	PULSATILLA NIGRICANS
Incontinence mainly during daytime.	Pale, delicate persons. Worse from motion.	FERRUM PHOSPHORICUM
After drinking water, especially cold water.	Worse for cold.	CANTHARIS VESICATORIA
INDIGESTION		
(See DYSPEPSIA)		
INFLUENZA		
Headache; sore throat; neuralgia, especially on right side; inflammation of ears. Sudden onset.	Better for warmth. Worse on lying down in the afternoon or at night. Lively, congenial persons may show temper when unwell.	ATROPA BELLADONNA
Chills up and down spine; red face; absence of thirst. Heavy eyelids.	Excitable, nervous persons. Better for open air. Worse about 10 a.m.	GELSEMIUM SEMPERVIRENS
Head pains; pains in limbs; cough, particularly on exertion.	Worse by movement and warmth. Dark-haired persons with dark complexion. Better from cold and rest.	BRYONIA ALBA
Fever; restlessness; pale; faintness.	Worse in dry, cold wind and in evening. Better in open air.	ACONITUM NAPELLUS
Headache; restlessness; cough.	Worse at night between 1 and 2 a.m. and in cold, wet weather. Tidy, fussy people.	ARSENICUM ALBUM
INSOMNIA		
(See SLEEPLESSNESS)		
ITCHING		
Better for scratching.	Worse in sunlight; shy, overweight persons.	CALCAREA CARBONICA

Symptoms/Sensations	Constitutions/Modalities	Remedies
Better for scratching, but causes burning sensation.	Persons who sweat easily with red orifices, for example, lips. Worse in morning.	SULFUR
Urge to scratch until skin bleeds; weeping eczema.	Worse at night, particularly before midnight.	GRAPHITES
With urticaria; due to allergies.	Worse for external irritants.	URTICA URENS

JAUNDICE

After a fright or extreme anger.	Worse for warmth and at 9 a.m.	CHAMOMILLA
With sharp pain in liver.	Better on laying on right side.	BRYONIA ALBA
With gallbladder pain.		CHELIDONIUM MAJUS
Malignant jaundice.	Better in dark room.	PHOSPHORUS
With itching skin; irritability; dyspepsia.	Better for warmth and sleep.	NUX VOMICA

JET LAG

With nausea and sickness; constipation.	Worse about 11 a.m. and when lying down.	IPECACUANHA
With intense headache; alcohol consumed during journey.	Better for sleep. Worse after meal.	NUX VOMICA
Nervousness; restlessness; homesickness; insomnia.	Worse in the morning and after coffee. Emotional, sensitive people.	IGNATIA AMARA
Near collapse; sensation of being displaced; fright from flight.	Worse for warmth and in the evening before midnight. Better in open air.	ACONITUM NAPELLUS
Physically exhausted; cramp; nosebleed.	Better for lying down; worse for cold.	ARNICA MONTANA

JOINTS, PAIN IN

With swelling, but little pain.	Worse for heat. Better for cold bathing.	APIS MELLIFICA
Cracking in joints on stretching.	Worse for damp weather	THUJA OCCIDENTALIS
Strained and rheumatic conditions.	Better for warmth.	RHUS TOXICODENDRON
Painful joints.	Women and children; worse by warmth; better for cold.	PULSATILLA NIGRICANS

Symptoms/Sensations	Constitutions/Modalities	Remedies
KNEES, PAIN IN		
Pain in knees; radiating pain.	Stout people. Worse on standing and exercise.	BERBERIS VULGARIS
"Housemaid's knee."	Worse about 10 a.m. and by heat. Better from cold bathing.	NATRUM MURIATICUM
Stiff and painful.	Worse by any movement and around 3 a.m. Sensitive to touch and motion.	BRYONIA ALBA
LARYNGITIS		
Acute laryngitis; red, flushed face; dry, painful larynx; spasmodic.	Worse at night and about 3 p.m.	ATROPA BELLADONNA
With restlessness, fever and anxiety; hacking cough; hoarseness.	Worse in evening and at night and in warm room. Better in open air.	ACONITUM NAPELLUS
Thick, stringy, yellow sputum; hard to clear.	Better for warmth.	KALI BICHROMICUM
Loose cough; hoarseness from singing, talking or shouting.	Worse in morning and in cold draft. Better for warmth and wrapping up head.	HEPAR SULFURIS
Barking cough; irritating, dry throat.	Better for warmth.	DROSERA ROTUNDIFOLIA
With irritating, dry throat and larynx; hard, dry cough; loss of voice; talking painful.	Worse during afternoon.	PHOSPHORUS
Chilly; sweating, poor circulation.	Worse for cold, damp air and in the evening.	CARBO VEGETABILIS
LEG CRAMP (See CRAMP)		
LIGAMENTS, PAIN IN		
From overexertion.	Better for warmth.	RHUS TOXICODENDRON
LIPS		
Dry lips; very thirsty.	Better for cold.	BRYONIA ALBA
Cracks in lips, particularly in center.	Better for cold.	NATRUM MURIATICUM
Swelling of upper lip; crack in center of lower lip; chapped lips. (See also HERPES)	Worse from cold, dry winds. Better for warmth.	HEPAR SULFURIS

Symptoms/Sensations	Constitutions/Modalities	Remedies
LUMBAGO		
From drafts; dry cold sensitive; sensation as if bruised.	Worse from touch, in evening and at night.	ACONITUM NAPELLUS
Backache with muscular pain; restlessness.		ACTAEA RACEMOSA
Stiffness; bruised, burning pain.	Better for gentle movement. Worse about 7 p.m.	RHUS TOXICODENDRON
Sensitive to touch; bruised feeling in back.	Worse when lying down, dry cold, and about 3 a.m.	BRYONIA ALBA
With urinary troubles or problems with rectum.	Worse on waking in morning.	BERBERIS VULGARIS
Deep-seated lumbago.	Worse for cold.	CALCAREA FLUORICA
Pain from blow or as if beaten; from getting chilled.	Worse during motion; better for rest and sleep.	NUX VOMICA
MEASLES		
In early stages of infection; restlessness; dry skin; catarrh-like symptoms; constant coughing at night.	Worse at night; better with bedclothes thrown off or in open air.	ACONITUM NAPELLUS
With sore throat; headache; swollen face.	Better for warmth; worse at night. Persons with reddish complexion.	ATROPA BELLADONNA
With catarrh and diarrhea.	Worse for warmth. Fair females with blue eyes, affectionate and shy.	PULSATILLA NIGRICANS
Hoarseness; stringy phlegm.		KALI BICHROMICUM
Conjunctivitis with much watering of the eyes; in early stages.	Worse for warmth; better from cold applications.	EUPHRASIA OFFICINALIS
With sore throat; difficulty in swallowing	Nervous people. Worse in morning.	GELSEMIUM SEMPERVIRENS
MENOPAUSE		
Sudden hot flashes with noticeable reddening of face; feeling of high temperature and considerable perspiration.	Active, friendly persons; sometimes violent temper. Better for warmth. Worse about 3 p.m.	ATROPA BELLADONNA

Symptoms/Sensations	Constitutions/Modalities	Remedies
Hot flashes, especially of face; sometimes nosebleeds and tendency to increase weight.	Cautious persons, slow to make decisions. Better in darkness. Worse before midnight.	GRAPHITES
Hot flashes with sensation of constriction around neck; fainting; left-sided pains.	Worse on waking in morning or for external pressure. Wants to be alone or put off things.	LACHESIS MUTUS
Hot sweats with sinking or dragging sensations.	Slim, dark-haired persons; easily depressed. Better in warm bed. Worse during morning.	SEPIA OFFICINALIS
Hot flashes with numbness; sinking sensations; nervousness; constipation; feeling of ball in throat.	Emotional, sensitive persons who may prefer to be alone. Worse in the mornings and after smoking or coffee. Better while eating.	IGNATIA AMARA
With restless; sleeplessness; sinking feeling.	Unhappy persons.	ACTAEA RACEMOSA

MENSTRUAL DISORDERS

Bad tempered at beginning; flow dark and clotted.	Worse for warmth.	CHAMOMILLA
Swelling of gums and cheeks; colic; bleeding ulcers.	Weepy moods; young women.	PHOSPHORUS
Faintness; sour taste in mouth.	Pale complexion, oily skin.	NATRUM MURIATICUM
Profuse periods; beginning early.	Worse at night and at full moon.	CALCAREA CARBONICA
Profuse periods; beginning early; burning in ovarian region; restlessness.	Worse after midnight. Better in warm room.	ARSENICUM ALBUM

(See also PREMENSTRUAL SYNDROME)

MENTAL EXHAUSTION

(See EXHAUSTION, MENTAL)

MOUTH ULCERS

With inflammation.	Better in open air and cold bathing.	NATRUM MURIATICUM
From injury.		HYPERICUM PERFORATUM

Symptoms/Sensations	Constitutions/Modalities	Remedies
With scruffy patches at corners of mouth; pimples on chin; yellow-based ulceration; gingivitis; gums and mouth painful to touch; tendency to bleed.	Worse for pressure. Better for wrapping up head.	HEPAR SULFURIS

MUMPS

In early stages; fever; thirst; anxiety; restlessness.	Better in open air. Worse in evening and at night.	ACONITUM NAPELLUS
If testicles are affected; orchitis.	Better for cold.	PULSATILLA NIGRICANS
When fever has subsided; burning in throat; loss of voice.	Worse at night and lying on right side.	MERCURIUS VIVUS

MUSCULAR PAIN

With stiff neck (torticollis); from a chill; numbness.	Worse on exposure to cold, dry wind and in warm room.	ACONITUM NAPELLUS
From dry cold.	Worse for any movement and at about 3 a.m.	BRYONIA ALBA
Pain in all limbs, moving about joints; pain in right foot and left arm; drawing in shoulders; cramp; nausea.	Worse in warm, damp weather and in the evening and for motion.	COLCHICUM AUTUMNALE
Pain in neck muscles; headache.	Better for warmth and sleep.	NUX VOMICA
Muscular pain from stab wound or injection.	Better for cold. Worse at night.	LEDUM PULUSTRE

(See also LUMBAGO, RHEUMATISM, NECK STIFFNESS.)

NAILS, PROBLEMS WITH

Easily cracked; rough; scaly.	Precise people.	ARSENICUM ALBUM
Brittle and powdery; rough; yellow color with white spots; striated lengthwise.		SILICA
Thick; ribbed surface; deformed, crumbly; inflamed at the matrix level.		GRAPHITES

Symptoms/Sensations	Constitutions/Modalities	Remedies
Brittle; associated with warts on fingers; striated across width of nails.	Dark-haired persons with dark skin.	THUJA OCCIDENTALIS
Pains under nails.	Better from hot applications.	SEPIA OFFICINALIS

NAUSEA

Constant, severe nausea with vomiting of food (green) or mucus; headache; hangover.	Worse in morning about 11 a.m. and after meals.	IPECACUANHA followed by NUX VOMICA
In pregnancy, with moist tongue.	Better in open air. Worse before midnight.	PULSATILLA NIGRICANS
With flatulence; digestive problems.	Worse for cold.	CALCAREA FLUORICA
On smelling cooking.	Worse by any movement and at night.	COLCHICUM AUTUMNALE
With burning pains; acid taste in mouth; exhaustion; nausea after drinking or eating.	Worse after midnight and for sight or smell of food. Craves coffee.	ARSENICUM ALBUM

(See also VOMITING)

NECK STIFFNESS

Severe stiff neck.	Worse by any movement.	PHYTOLACCA DECANDRA
From draft or chill; painful in nape of neck extending down into the shoulder; numbness; anxiety.	Worse on movement or exposure to dry cold. Better in open air.	ACONITUM NAPELLUS
With rheumatic pain; stiffness in neck and back muscles; spine sensitivity; pain moves down back; during menses.	Worse from touch or motion.	ACTAEA RACEMOSA
Paralysis, drawing in shoulders.	Worse by movement and in the evening and at night.	COLCHICUM AUTUMNALE
With hoarseness; swollen glands in neck.	Worse for cold.	CALCAREA CARBONICA
At onset.	Elderly persons. Worse by first movement. Better for firmly applied pressure.	BRYONIA ALBA

Symptoms/Sensations	Constitutions/Modalities	Remedies
After exertion; by false movement.	Worse for least touch, motion, rest and damp cold. Better with head held low.	ARNICA MONTANA

NEURALGIA

Facial neuralgia.	Especially on the right side of face.	ATROPA BELLADONNA
Facial neuralgia from cold drafts; with numbness.	Worse in dry, cold wind and in evening. Better in open air.	ACONITUM NAPELLUS
Pains like electric shocks in limbs, especially sciatic plexus.		MAGNESIUM PHOSPHORICUM
Pure neuralgia pain with restlessness; intermittent pain.	Worse in morning and by cold applications. Better by exercise, at night, and by warmth.	ARSENICUM ALBUM
With nervousness; intolerable pain; great thirst; toothache; earache.	Worse at night and by warmth.	CHAMOMILLA
In bones; with swelling.		PHYTOLACCA DECANDRA
Intercostal neuralgia.	Worse from touch and from motion.	CHELIDONIUM MAJUS
Sudden pain.	Especially on right side of head and face. Worse for movement or touch and 4 to 8 p.m.	LYCOPODIUM CLAVATUM

NOSEBLEED

With red face and throbbing headache.	Worse 10 p.m. to midnight	ATROPA BELLADONNA
Frequent nosebleeds; profuse bleeding; tightness in bridge of nose.	Worse in warm air.	HAMAMELIS VIRGINIANA
From a blow to the nose; after fit of coughing; sore nose; cold feeling.	Worse for cold. Better for head held low or lying down.	ARNICA MONTANA
Bright red blood.	On rising in the morning.	BRYONIA ALBA
Clotted blood.	On rising in the morning.	NUX VOMICA
Frequent with profuse bleeding; sudden onset.	Worse during afternoon.	PHOSPHORUS
Recurrent bleeding; sneezing.	Elderly persons. Worse about 4 to 5 p.m.	CARBO VEGETABILIS

Symptoms/Sensations	Constitutions/Modalities	Remedies
Before or accompanying biliousness.		CHELIDONIUM MAJUS
Recurrent bleeding; no apparent cause; with feverish illness.	Children. Worse for pressure, touch, motion and at night. Better from cold applications.	FERRUM PHOSPHORICUM

NUMBNESS

With tingling in hands; pain down left arm; shooting pains; icy cold hands and feet.	Worse in warm room and in evening.	ACONITUM NAPELLUS
Numbness on one side, particularly right side; creeping feeling in hands and feet; cramp in calves.	Worse in cold, wet weather and on right side. Better for heat.	ARSENICUM ALBUM
Numbness in heel on walking.	Worse in the morning. Better for change in position.	IGNATIA AMARA
With tingling and exhaustion.	Worse about 10 to 11 a.m. Better for cold.	NATRUM MURIATICUM
With numbness in hands.	Worse when grasping.	CHAMOMILLA
Numbness in finger tips.	Worse sunset to sunrise and for movement.	COLCHICUM AUTUMNALE

OBESITY

(Note: Proper diet and regular exercise are recommended.)

With enlarged glands; constipation.	Fair people who feel chilly.	CALCAREA CARBONICA
With small boils.	Better after eating. Craving for acid foods, wine and strong-tasting foods.	HEPAR SULFURIS
With red face; dyspepsia.		FERRUM PHOSPHORICUM
With skin disease.		GRAPHITES

OFFENSIVE BREATH

(See BREATH, BAD)

OTITIS

Acute pain in ear; throbbing, pulsating sensations; inflammation of eustachian tube; noises.	Worse at night, especially 4 p.m. to 6 p.m. and touch.	FERRUM PHOSPHORICUM

Symptoms/Sensations	Constitutions/Modalities	Remedies
Inflammation of external orifice; swelling; sensation as if drops of water in ear.	Worse for music and noise, and in evening.	ACONITUM NAPELLUS
PAINS		
From blows, injuries (usually traumatic); limbs aching as if beaten.	Prefers to be alone. Worse for cold, motion and touch. Better for lying down.	ARNICA MONTANA
Bone pains.	Worse about 3 p.m.	ATROPA BELLADONNA
Severe, tearing pains; spasmodic pains; cramps.	Better for pressure. Worse from contact and vomiting.	CUPRUM METALLICUM
Rheumatic pains; neuralgia; pain at root of nose; headache on waking.	Worse after sleep and on left side. Better for warm applications.	LACHESIS MUTUS
Congestive pains.	Worse on waking, on left side, and between 4 and 8 p.m.	LYCOPODIUM CLAVATUM
Sudden pains; right-sided pains.	Worse between 4 and 8 p.m.	MAGNESIA PHOSPHORICUM
Rheumatic pains.	Worse about 7 p.m.	RHUS TOXICODENDRON
Shooting pains.	Worse after movement or in cold and damp.	ACTAEA RACEMOSA
PERSPIRATION		
After walking; sweating at night; on head and chest; from excitement.	People with pale, sickly complexion. Worse for hot food or drink and in warm, wet weather.	PHOSPHORUS
Sweaty palms; sweating after midnight.	Worse 1 to 2 p.m. and for food.	ARSENICUM ALBUM
Hot, sweaty feet.	Persons subject to skin problems.	SULFUR
Offensive, smelly, cold, sweating feet.	People with delicate, pale skin. Worse in winter.	SILICA
Sweating forehead and head.	Worse at 3 a.m. Children.	CALCAREA CARBONICA

(See also BODY ODOR)

PHARYNGITIS
(See SORE THROAT)

PILES
(See HEMORRHOIDS)

Symptoms/Sensations	Constitutions/Modalities	Remedies
PIMPLES (See ACNE)		
PREMENSTRUAL SYNDROME (Premenstrual Tension)		(Note: Regular meals and regular exercise recommended.)
Perspiration, especially the head; vertigo; headache; chilliness; tender breasts; period profuse and early.	Worse at night and about 2 p.m. Quiet, shy, sensitive women; subject to depression.	CALCAREA CARBONICA
Period too late or too long; cramps which may extend into chest, fingers, legs and toes; nausea.	Worse at night.	CUPRUM METALLICUM
Anguish; anxiety; fluid retention and heaviness of breasts; cannot bear clothing; apathetic; fainting spell; hot flashes.	Slim, pale-complected women who are conscientious with keen intellect. Worse after sleep and in spring.	LACHESIS MUTUS
Bad tempered; melancholic; bloating urinary symptoms; cries easily.	Worse at night; aversion to bread. Slim-faced women who prefer company. Better for warmth.	LYCOPODIUM CLAVATUM
Sneezing; allergies; herpes; hypochondriacal.	Laughing or weepy. Worse about 10 to 11 a.m.	NATRUM MURIATICUM
Changeable symptoms; painful breasts; delayed period; ringing in ears; greenish nasal or vaginal discharge.	Timid, tearful, blonde, fair-complected women and girls. Worse about 4 p.m.	PULSATILLA NIGRICANS
Depressed; irritable; tired feeling, morose.	Slim, dark-haired women, below average height. Better in warm bed and in the evening.	SEPIA OFFICINALIS
PSORIASIS		
General psoriasis; thickened skin; burning; itching; restlessness.	Pale, slim, sensitive, precise intelligent persons. Worse after midnight and in wet weather.	ARSENICUM ALBUM
General psoriasis.	Young girls.	CUPRUM METALLICUM

Symptoms/Sensations	Constitutions/Modalities	Remedies
With neuralgia; debility; intermittent pain.	Older, precise persons. Worse between 1 and 2 p.m. and after midnight. Worse for cold and for rapid movement. Better for warmth and warm drinks.	ARSENICUM ALBUM
Pain on right side.	Worse from 4 to 8 p.m., by touch or lying on the right side.	LYCOPODIUM CLAVATUM
Pain on right side; like lightning.	Worse on coughing. Better for warmth.	MAGNESIA PHOSPHORICUM
Limbs giving way; pain as if from blows.	Worse from cold and on lying down.	RUTA GRAVEOLENS
Chronic sciatica; burning, tearing pains.	Better for heat and movement. Worse when resting.	RHUS TOXICODENDRON
Pain on right side.	Better lying down. Worse after sleep and from pressure.	LACHESIS MUTUS

SCURF

(see DANDRUFF)

SEXUAL PROBLEMS

Marked anxiety and fear of intercourse; headaches; loss of erection when intercourse attempted; shriveled genitals.	Worse by hot room and at night. Impulsive, nervous people. Better for cold and pressure.	ARGENTUM NITRICUM
Variable frigidity; back pain and tired feeling during menstruation.	Shy, fair haired, tearful young women. Worse for heat and warm bedroom.	PULSATILLA NIGRICANS
From injury or blow to genital area.	Better bending head backward. Worse when genitals cold.	HYPERICUM PERFORATUM
Frigidity; changeable moods; disappointment with sexual experience.	Moody women who tend to be uncommunicative. Worse in morning.	IGNATIA AMARA
Tenderness, burning, soreness of vagina with cutting pain during intercourse. Smarting and neuralgia in testicles.	Women with tendency for urinary complaints.	BERBERIS VULGARIS
With general nervous depression; irritability; constipation; drinking alcohol.	Slim, dark persons. Better for sleep. Worse before 3 a.m.	NUX VOMICA

Symptoms/Sensations	Constitutions/Modalities	Remedies
Pain in genitals affects intercourse.	Cautious persons; better in dark. Worse for cold and before midnight.	GRAPHITES
Anxiety about sexual performance; dyspepsia; long standing impotence.	Insecure persons; pale complexion; slim-faced. Worse for cold.	LYCOPODIUM CLAVATUM
Itching and redness of genitals.	Likes alcohol. Worse for warmth.	SULFUR

SHINGLES

(See HERPES)

SHOCK

| With fever; from fright; immediately after an accident; collapse; sensations as if in dream. | Worse for music and warmth. | ACONITUM NAPELLUS |
| In long term; after traumatic injuries; sudden bad news (for example, financial loss). | Prefers to be alone. Better for lying down. | ARNICA MONTANA |

SHOULDER PAIN

| Hot, red, swollen; pain radiates into arm; affects right shoulder. | Much worse for any movement, at night, and cold. | FERRUM PHOSPHORICUM |

SINUS OBSTRUCTION

With pain, especially in frontal sinuses.	Worse on bending forward.	ATROPA BELLADONNA
Yellow, stringy catarrh.	Better for warmth.	KALI BICHROMICUM
Intermittent nasal obstruction causing pain above the eyes.	Better for cold. Worse about 4 p.m.	PULSATILLA NIGRICANS
Tearing head pains; nausea.	Worse about 10 to 11 a.m. Better for cold.	NATRUM MURIATICUM
Pain as if in bones around sinuses; begins at back of head and settles over eyes.	Better for warmth. Worse in winter.	SILICA

SLEEPLESSNESS

| Through excitement; irritable; teething; spoiled child; sleeps with eyes open. | Particularly children. | CHAMOMILLA |
| Sleeplessness at night and after eating; restless; dreams; fearful. | Tall, slim people. Worse for cold food. | PHOSPHORUS |

Symptoms/Sensations	Constitutions/Modalities	Remedies
Nightmares; sudden waking; agitated.	Better for warmth.	SILICA
Sleeplessness; depression; with uterine infection.	Nervous, confused persons.	ACTAEA RACEMOSA
Tired but cannot sleep; anxiety dreams; jerking limbs; throbbing headache.	Better for warmth. Worse for cold.	ATROPA BELLADONNA
Restless in bed; anxiety dreams; palpitation.	Better for warmth. Worse at midnight.	RHUS TOXICODENDRON
No exact cause; light sleep.	Easily woken up; better for cold.	
Light sleeping; yawning; very nervous; restlessness; dreams; following bereavement.	Worse in the early morning. Dislikes tobacco smoke.	IGNATIA AMARA with CHAMOMILLA
Restlessness; tossing and turning; high temperature; nightmares.	Worse at midnight or in warm bedroom. Particularly elderly people.	ACONITUM NAPELLUS
Overactive mind at night; worry; depression.	Better in early hours of morning. Slim-faced persons.	LYCOPODIUM CLAVATUM

SORE THROAT

Chronic, dry, rough, sore throat; cannot swallow.	Worse at night and in cold, damp weather.	PHYTOLACCA DECANDRA
With swelling, rawness; dropping of mucus from back of nose.		HYDRASTIS CANADENSIS
Nervous sore throat; pain on swallowing; "lump" in throat.	Worse when swallowing liquids; better when swallowing food.	IGNATIA AMARA
Nervous sore throat; throat irritation; choking; coughing; "lump" in throat; very painful.	Worse on left side of throat, for slightest pressure and after sleep.	LACHESIS MUTUS
From talking too much or shouting; raw, sore feeling.	Worse for cold and in the morning.	ARNICA MONTANA
From exposure to cold; at the onset of sore throat; thirsty; constricted feeling; stinging sensation.	Worse in warm room, in evening and from cold, dry winds.	ACONITUM NAPELLUS
With difficulty in swallowing.	Worse in warm room. Better in open air.	GELSEMIUM SEMPERVIRENS

Symptoms/Sensations	Constitutions/Modalities	Remedies
With pus on tonsils or throat walls; desire to swallow.	Sensitive to hot and cold. Worse at night and for hot drinks. Throat worse on right side.	MERCURIUS VIVUS

SPRAINS

Painful sprains, particularly wrists and ankles; bruising; over exertion.	Better for warmth and lying down. Worse for damp cold.	ARNICA MONTANA
Residual stiffness and rheumatic pain from a sprain; sprains of joints or tendons.	Worse at night. Worse on initial movement but better on continued movement.	RHUS TOXICODENDRON
Sprains in wrists or ankles; bruised pain in bones and ligaments.	Worse for cold.	RUTA GRAVEOLENS
Residual weakness; later stages of sprains	Worse for cold. Better for warmth.	CALCAREA CARBONICA

STINGS

Insect stings, particularly bee or wasp stings. Painful; red; swollen; in state of near collapse; sore; sensitive.	Worse from heat and pressure. Better in open air and cold bathing.	APIS MELLIFICA
Bee stings; burning; itching. (See also BITES)	Worse from water and cool, moist air.	URTICA URENS

STRESS

(See ANXIETY, EXHAUSTION, DIARRHEA, FAINTING, HEADACHES, PAIN, SLEEPLESSNESS)

STYES

At onset. Eyelids stick together on waking.	Worse for warmth and in morning.	PULSATILLA NIGRICANS
Recurring styes.	Worse in cold wind.	HEPAR SULFURIS
With honey-colored exudate.	Worse before midnight.	GRAPHITES

SUNBURN

Preventive.		NATRUM MURIATICUM
Edema; pink skin; sharp, burning pain.	Better by heat.	URTICA URENS

Symptoms/Sensations	Constitutions/Modalities	Remedies
Scalding, violent pain in bladder; frequent urination in small quantities; inflammation.	Worse from touch and when urinating.	CANTHARIS VESICATORIA
Dribbling on coughing, passing wind or laughing.	Worse at night. Fair haired, blue-eyed persons, especially young women.	PULSATILLA NIGRICANS

(See also INCONTINENCE)

URTICARIA

Chronic or recurring urticaria.	Worse from air. Better from warmth.	HEPAR SULFURIS
Persistent urticaria.	Worse between 4 and 8 p.m.	LYCOPODIUM CLAVATUM
Most cases; stinging; itching; irritation; violent pruritis.	Worse for touch and water application. Better by heat.	URTICA URENS
After ingestion of spoiled foods.	Better by heat.	ARSENICUM ALBUM
After ingestion of fatty foods.	Worse about 4 p.m.	PULSATILLA NIGRICANS

(See also ITCHING)

VARICOSE VEINS

With hemorrhoids; tendency to ulceration; very sore.	For alleviation. Worse during day and in warm moist air.	HAMAMELIS VIRGINIANA
With chilliness; cramps.	Overweight persons.	CALCAREA CARBONICA
Associated poor circulation.		CARBO VEGETABILIS

VERTIGO

Tendency to fall forward.	Dark-haired people. Worse from warmth. Worse in bed or on rising.	BRYONIA ALBA ATROPA BELLADONNA
With travel sickness.		COCCULUS INDICUS
With trembling and giddiness.	Nervous people. Worse in morning. Better in open air.	GELSEMIUM SEMPERVIRENS
With headache and constipation	Worse when lying down.	NATRUM MURIATICUM

VOMITING

Simple vomiting; nausea; salivation; diarrhea.	Worse about 11 a.m.	IPECACUANHA

Symptoms/Sensations	Constitutions/Modalities	Remedies
Vomiting of cold water.	Worse during afternoon.	PHOSPHORUS
With burning pains or irritability in stomach; gastritis; diarrhea; coldness in hands and feet; thirst; vomiting of blood or bile.	Worse for sight or smell of food and after eating or drinking.	ARSENICUM ALBUM
From overeating or excess alcohol.	Worse 2 to 3 hours after meals. Better for warmth.	NUX VOMICA

WARTS

General warts; bleed easily; red eczema between eyebrows.	Use mother tincture locally. Persons who perspire easily and gain excess weight easily; worries at night.	THUJA OCCIDENTALIS
Numerous small warts; warts on hands; itching; inflammation; stinging.		CALCAREA CARBONICA
On palms of hands.		RUTA GRAVEOLENS
Horny warts.		GRAPHITES

WEAKNESS

With irritability; loss of appetite; constipation.	Worse for cold foods.	NUX VOMICA
	Overweight children.	CALCAREA CARBONICA
	Slim, rickety children. Worse about 2 p.m.	SILICA
	Worse in the morning and when lying in bed.	PULSATILLA NIGRICANS
Irritable weakness; restlessness; debility.	After eating. Worse at night. Better for warmth.	ARSENICUM ALBUM
	After walking.	RUTA GRAVEOLENS
	Worse in the evening.	NATRUM MURIATICUM
	Worse during periods and during morning.	SEPIA OFFICINALIS

WHITLOWS

	In early stages.	SILICA
Prickling, tingling with extended blue or purple coloration.	Worse after sleep. Better for warm applications.	LACHESIS MUTUS

Symptoms/Sensations	Constitutions/Modalities	Remedies
With much throbbing.	Worse at night with loss of sleep, from cold air. Better for warmth.	HEPAR SULFURIS
Finger is hot and throbbing.	Worse about 3 p.m.	ATROPA BELLADONNA

WHOOPING COUGH

Preventive.	Worse after midnight.	DROSERA ROTUNDIFOLIA
Spasmodic fits of coughing; vomiting after coughing.	Worse about 11 a.m.	IPECACUANHA
Spasms; cramps.	Better for drinking cold water.	CUPRUM METALLICUM
Spasmodic coughing; rattling in chest.	Fair people. Worse for cold. Sensitive to slightest draft. Better after eating.	HEPAR SULFURIS

WOUNDS

Cuts and abrasions; superficial burns and scalds; yellowness.	Sensitive to open air.	CALENDULA OFFICINALIS
Infected wounds.	Worse for cold. Wants wound to be covered.	HEPAR SULFURIS
Crushed fingers or toes, affecting nerve endings; puncture wounds.	Worse for cold, exposure and touch.	HYPERICUM PERFORATUM
Puncture wounds, for example, injections, needle injury or insect bites; redness; mottling; throbbing pain. (See also FRACTURES, BRUISES)	Robust people with redness of face. Symptoms generally worse for heat and at night. Better from cold.	LEDUM PALUSTRE

YAWNING

After dinner; apprehensive; poor memory.	Worse between 4 and 8 p.m. from heat and warm room. Better for motion.	LYCOPODIUM CLAVATUM
Frequent yawning and sleepiness, as if been awake all night; lethargic; vertigo.	Worse for motion, change of weather and in morning.	CHELIDONIUM MAJUS
Frequent yawning after sleeping; yawning while eating; tearful.	Emotional people who are introspective. Worse in morning, after meals and smoking. Better while eating and for change in position.	IGNATIA AMARA

COMMON HOMEOPATHIC REMEDIES AND THERAPEUTIC INDICES

1. ACONITUM NAPELLUS

Abbreviated Name: ACONITE
Common Name: Monkshood
Source: Plant
Introduced by Hahnemann et al. in *Fragmenta di Viribus Medicamentorum*, published in Leipzig in 1805.
The mother tincture is prepared from the whole plant.

Modalities

Symptoms better in the open air.

Symptoms worse when lying on affected side, when rising from bed, in warm rooms, dry, cold winds and in evening, particularly before midnight.

Antidotes

Belladonna; Berberis; Coffea; Sulfur; Nux Vomica.

Constitutional Factors

Especially active for young people, especially girls with dark hair, dark eyes, fearful, prefer sedentary life.

Therapeutic Index:

Alcoholism	Excitement	Neck Stiffness
Anger	Fainting	Neuralgia
Bereavement	Fear	Numbness
Bites	Hoarseness	Otitis
Bronchitis	Influenza	Rheumatism
Colds	Jet Lag	Sciatica
Concussion	Laryngitis	Shock
Conjunctivitis	Lumbago	Sleeplessness
Cough	Measles	Sore throat
Croup	Menopausal Disorders	Sunstroke
Earache	Mumps	Tonsilitis
	Muscular Pain	

2. ACTAEA RACEMOSA

Abbreviated Name: ACTAEA RAC.
Common Name: Baneberry
Source: Plant
The mother tincture is prepared from the root of the plant.

Modalities

Symptoms better for warmth.

Symptoms worse in the morning, cold and damp conditions, from movement and during periods.

Antidotes

None listed.

Constitutional Factors

Especially for people who are active, particularly women.

Therapeutic index:

Backache	Headache	Neck Stiffness
Depression	Hysteria	Pains
Emotional Problems	Lumbago	Sleeplessness
	Menopausal Disorders	

3. APIS MELLIFICA

Abbreviated Name: APIS MEL.
Common Name: Honey Bee
Source: Animal
The mother tincture is prepared from the whole, live honey bee.

Modalities

Symptoms better in open air, cold bathing, removing clothes, walking or movement and sitting erect.

Symptoms worse for heat, touch, pressure, after sleeping, heated rooms, getting wet and on the right side.

Antidotes

Cantharis; Ipecac.; Lachesis; Ledum; Nat. Mur.

Constitutional Factors

Especially active for women, children and girls who may be awkward, though generally careful.

Therapeutic index:

Abscesses	Bursitis	Feet Discomfort
Ankles, Swollen	Coccyx Pain	Pain in Joints
Arthritis, Acute	Cystitis	Stings
Bites	Diarrhea	Toothache
Boils	Dry Mouth	Urinary Disorders

4. ARGENTUM NITRICUM

Abbreviated Name: ARGENT. NIT.
Common Name: Silver Nitrate
Source: Plant
Soluble white, rhombic-shaped crystal with formula $AgNo_3$.

Modalities

Symptoms better for fresh air, pressure, bathing in cold water.

Symptoms worse for cold food, cold air, warmth, at night, after eating, particularly sweet foods, during periods, exceptional mental exertion and on the left side.

Antidotes

Lycopodium; Nat. Mur.; Phosphorus; Rhus Tox.; Sepia; Sulfur; Pulsatilla; Merc. Viv.

Constitutional Factors

Especially active for nervous, impulsive, irritable people who desire candies. Old, thin, scrawny people.

Therapeutic Index:

Acidity	Dyspepsia	Sexual Problems
Acute Arthritis	Emotional Problems	Tongue Disorders
Apprehension	Fear	
Conjunctivitis	Flatulence	
Diarrhea	Headache	

5. ARNICA MONTANA

Abbreviated Name: ARNICA
Common Name: Mountain Arnica
Source: Plant
Introduced by Hahnemann et al. in *Fragmenta di Viribus Medicamentorum*, published in Leipzig in 1805.

Modalities

Symptoms better for contact and motion.

Symptoms worse for touch, motion, rest, damp conditions and wine.

Antidotes

Aconite; Camphor; China; Ignatia; Ipecac.

Constitutional Factors

Especially active for nervous women with lively expression and red faces, who remain affected from mechanical injuries long ago.

Therapeutic Index:

Acne Rosacea	Concussion	Nosebleed
Acute Arthritis	Cramp	Pains
Backache	Distended Abdomen	Rheumatism
Bad Breath	Exhaustion, Physical	Shock
Boils	Foot Discomfort	Sore Throat
Bruises	Hair Loss	Sprains
Carbuncles	Hoarseness	Trauma
	Neck Stiffness	

6. ARSENICUM ALBUM

Abbreviated Name: ARSEN. ALB.
Common Name: Arsenious Oxide
Source: Mineral
Insoluble, white powder of formula As_2O_3.

Modalities

Symptoms better for heat and warm drinks.
Symptoms worse for cold, cold drinks, wet weather, and between 1 a.m. and 2 a.m.

Antidotes

Carbo Veg.; China; Nux Vomica; Hepar Sulf.; Euphrasia; Ipecac.; Camphor; Kali Bich.; Veratrum Alb.

Constitutional Factors

Especially active in irritable people who are restless, sensitive and may fear death.

Therapeutic Index:

Acne Rosacea	Fainting	Perspiration
Alcoholism	Fear	Psoriasis
Apprehension	Gingivitis	Ringworm
Backache	Hay Fever	Sciatica
Blisters	Herpes	Thirst
Boils	Influenza	Tongue Disorders
Breathing Difficulty	Menstrual Disorders	Ulcers
Colds	Nail Problems	Urticaria
Colitis	Nausea	Vomiting
Dyspepsia	Neuralgia	Weakness
	Numbness	

7. ATROPA BELLADONNA

Abbreviated Name: BELLADONNA
Common Name: Deadly Nightshade
Source: Plant
Introduced by Hahnemann et al. in *Fragmenta di Viribus Medicamentorum* in 1805, the name is derived from the usage of the juice of its berries during the 14th Century as a cosmetic, hence, *bella donna*—beautiful lady.

Modalities

Symptoms better for sitting erect, standing and in warm room.
Symptoms worse for touch, motion, drafts, bright lights, noise, jar, lying down, about 3 p.m. and 10 p.m. to midnight.

Antidotes

Aconite; Merc. Viv.; Sabadilla; Camphor; Hepar Sulf.

Constitutional Factors

Especially active for people with hot, red skin, flushed face and glaring eyes. Bilious people who are lively and entertaining. Women have light hair, blue eyes and fine complexion, sensitive and nervous.

Therapeutic Index:

Abscesses	Earache	Neuralgia
Acne	Excitement	Nosebleed
Acne Rosacea	Fear	Pains
Aggressiveness	Giddiness	Salivation Deficiency
Bronchitis	Grinding of teeth	Sinusitis
Candida Infection	Headache	Sleeplessness
Carbuncles	Incontinence	Sunburn
Chilblains	Influenza	Sunstroke
Conjunctivitis	Laryngitis	Thirst
Cough	Measles	Tongue Disorders
Depression	Menopausal Problems	Whitlows

8. BERBERIS VULGARIS

Abbreviated Name: BERBERIS
Common Name: Barberry
Source: Plant

Modalities

Symptoms worse for standing, motion or jarring and rest.

Antidotes

Belladonna; Camphor.

Constitutional Factors

Especially active for gregarious persons.

Therapeutic Index:

Bilious Attack	Knee Pain	Rheumatism
Bladder Disorders	Lumbago	Sexual Problems
Hemorrhoids		Urinary Disorders

9. BRYONIA ALBA

Abbreviated Name: BRYONIA
Common Name: Wild Hops
Source: Plant
The mother tincture is prepared from the root of the plant.
One of the original remedies proved by Hahnemann.

Modalities

Symptoms better for lying down, particularly on affected side, pressure, rest, cold and cold food.

Symptoms worse for motion, exertion, warmth, hot weather, touch and about 3 a.m. or 9 p.m.

Antidotes

Aconite; Antim. Tart; Belladonna; Berberis; Carbo Veg.; Nux Vom.; Phos; Pulsatilla; Sulfur.

Constitutional Factors

Especially active for dark-haired people with dark complexion, slender, irritable, nervous and prone to anger and bilious attacks.

Therapeutic Index:

Abdominal Pains	Constipation	Jaundice
Abscesses	Cough	Lip Problems
Bilious Attack	Dry Mouth	Lumbago
Bronchitis	Eczema	Muscular Pain
Chestiness	Giddiness	Neck Stiffness
Colds	Hair Loss	Nosebleed
	Headache	
	Influenza	

10. CALCAREA CARBONICA

Abbreviated Name: CALC. CARB.
Common Name: Calcium Carbonate
Source: Mineral
Originally prepared by Hahnemann from the ground, middle layer of oyster shell as impure form of calcium carbonate, $CaCO_3$.

Modalities

Symptoms better for dry weather and lying on affected side. Symptoms worse for cold air, wet weather, cold water, mental or physical exertion, standing, water and about 2 p.m.

Antidotes

Bryonia; Camphor; Ipecac.; China; Nux Vom.; Sepia; Sulfur.

Constitutional Factors:

Especially active for people with blond hair, pale complexion and blue eyes. Sensitive, shy, easily embarrassed and easily tired.

Therapeutic Index:

Abdomen, Distended	Itching	Ringworm
Adenoids	Menstrual Disorders	Sprains
Appetite, Craving	Neck Stiffness	Teething
Appetite, Loss of	Obesity	Toothache
Backache	Perspiration	Varicose Veins
Debility	Premenstrual Syndrome	Warts
Giddiness	Rheumatism	Weakness

11. CALCAREA FLUORICA

Abbreviated Name: CALC. FLUOR.
Common Name: Calcium Fluoride
Source: Mineral
Soluble, white powder as naturally occurring fluorspar of formula CaF_2.

Modalities

Symptoms better for heat and gentle movement.
Symptoms worse for rest, damp weather or changes in weather.

Antidotes

None listed.

Therapeutic Index:

Backache	Catarrh	Uterine Infections
Burning Pain	Gout	Lumbago, Deep Seated
	Head Cold	

12. CALCAREA PHOSPHORICA

Abbreviated Name: CALC. PHOS.
Common Name: Calcium Phosphate
Source: Mineral
Insoluble, white powder of formula $Ca_3(PO_4)_2$, from bones.

Modalities

Symptoms better for warm, dry summer weather.
Symptoms worse for cold, damp, melting snow and mental effort.

Antidotes

None listed.

Constitutional Factors

Especially active for anemic, thin, dark-haired people with dark eyes. Emaciated children with feeble digestion.

Therapeutic Index:

Acute Disease (After)	Debility	Throbbing Headache
Adenoids	Exhaustion	Toothache
	Fractures	
	Gingivitis	

13. CALENDULA OFFICINALIS

Abbreviated Name: CALENDULA
Common Name: Marigold
Source: Plant
The mother tincture is prepared from the fresh, flowering plant cut just above the roots.

Modalities

Symptoms worse for damp weather.

Antidotes

Arnica

Constitutional Factors

Especially suited for depressed, easily frightened, irritable people who dislike cold weather.

Therapeutic Index:

Chapped Skin	Cuts	Ulcers
Candida Infection	Sores	Wounds
	Trauma	

14. CANTHARIS VESICATORIA

Abbreviated Name: CANTHARIS
Common Name: Spanish Fly
Source: Animal
The mother tincture is prepared from dried, powdered insect.

Modalities

Symptoms better for rubbing.
Symptoms worse for urinating, touch, drinking cold water, food, tobacco or coffee, erections.

Antidotes

Aconite; Camphor; Pulsatilla.

Constitutional Factors

Especially active for people who are physically oversensitive.

Therapeutic Index:

Bladder Disorders	Burns	Incontinence
Blisters	Colitis	Tongue Disorders
	Cystitis	
	Dandruff	

15. CARBO VEGETABILIS

Abbreviated Name: CARBO VEG.
Common Name: Wood Charcoal
Source: Plant/Mineral
Residue from controlled burning of beech or birch wood, principally black carbon with traces of mineral salts.

Modalities

Symptoms better for cold.
Symptoms worse for warm, damp weather, fatty food, open air, singing and about 4 to 5 pm.

Antidotes

Arsen Alb.; Coffea; Camphor; Lachesis.

Constitutional Factors

Especially active for sluggish, fat, lazy people who are embarrassed in company, dislike darkness and prone to sudden loss of memory. People who have never fully recovered from exhausting effects of previous illness or injury.

Therapeutic Index:

Acne	Belching	Leg Cramp
Angina	Collapse	Nosebleed
Anus Disorders	Dyspepsia	Saliva, Excess
Apprehension	Flatulence	Varicose Veins
	Headache	

16. CHAMOMILLA

Common Name: Wild Chamomile
Source: Plant
Introduced by Hahnemann in his book, *Fragmenta di Viribus Medicamentorum* in 1805.

The mother tincture is prepared from the whole plant. Often called the Children's Remedy.

Modalities

Symptoms better for being carried or rocked, warm, wet weather.

Symptoms worse for heat, anger, tantrums, open air, at night and about 9 a.m.

Constitutional Factors

Especially active for people, especially children, with light-brown hair who are nervous, excitable and sensitive to coffee or narcotics. Peevish, restless children who "cry uncontrollably, wants this and that, and when given anything, it is refused or knocked away" (Hahnemann).

Therapeutic Index:

Anger	Earache	Menstrual Disorders
Candida Infection	Excitement	Numbness
Diarrhea	Feet Discomfort	Sleeplessness
Dyspeps:a	Flatulence	Teething
	Jaundice	

17. CHELIDONIUM MAJUS

Abbreviated Name: CHELIDONIUM
Common Name: Greater Celandine
Source: Plant

Modalities

Symptoms better for pressure.

Symptoms worse for motion, touch, change of weather, about 4 to 5 a.m. and on the right side.

Antidotes

Aconite: Chamomilla; Coffea.

Constitutional Factors

Especially active for people with light complexion, fair hair, thin, irritable, prone to gastric and abdominal problems.

Therapeutic Index:

Bad Breath	Headache	Nosebleed
Bilious Attack	Jaundice	Yawning
	Neuralgia	

18. COLCHICUM AUTUMNALE

Abbreviated Name: COLCHICUM
Common Name: Autumn Crocus
Source: Plant
The mother tincture is prepared from the juice of the corn lifted from the ground in Spring.

Modalities

Symptoms better for stooping and sleep.

Symptoms worse for mental exertion, loss of sleep, at night and motion.

Antidotes

Belladonna; Camphor; Cocculus; Ledum, Nux Vomica; Pulsatilla; Spigelia.

Constitutional Factors

Especially active for people who are robust, gouty, very sensitive to noise, odors, other people's actions.

Therapeutic Index:

Colitis	Feet Discomfort	Numbness
Cramp	Gout	Rheumatism
Diarrhea	Muscular Pain	Travel Sickness
	Neck Stiffness	

19. CUPRUM METALLICUM

Abbreviated Name: CUPRUM MET.
Common Name: Copper Metal
Source: Mineral
Pure, reddish powdered metal (trituration).

Modalities

Symptoms better for drinking cold water, nausea, perspiration.
Symptoms worse for cold air, vomiting, contact and at night.

Antidotes

Belladonna; Camphor; China; Cocculus.

Constitutional Factors

Especially active for anxious people who are easily tired.

Therapeutic Index:

Asthma	Pains	Sunstroke
Cramp	Premenstrual Syndrome	Whooping Cough

20. DROSERA ROTUNDIFOLIA

Abbreviated Name: DROSERA
Common Name: Sundew
Source: Plant
Originally proved by Hahnemann et al. and included in his *Fragmenta di Viribus Medicamentorum* in 1805, and later in *Materia Medica Pura*. The mother tincture is prepared from the whole plant.

Modalities

Symptoms better for keeping erect.
Symptoms worse for lying down, drinking, being too warm in bed and from midnight to 3 a.m.

Antidotes

Camphor.

Therapeutic Index:

Constipation	Laryngitis	Whooping Cough

21. EUPHRASIA OFFICINALIS

Abbreviated Name: EUPHRASIA
Common Name: Eyebright

Source: Plant

The mother tincture is prepared from the whole, fresh plant.

Modalities

Symptoms better for coffee and at night.

Symptoms worse for warm rooms, light and in the evening.

Antidotes

Causticum; Camphor; Pulsatilla.

Constitutional Factors

Especially active for indolent or depressed people who dislike talking.

Therapeutic Index:

Colds	Conjunctivitis	Measles
	Hay fever	

22. FERRUM PHOSPHORICUM

Abbreviated Name: FERRUM PHOS.
Common Name: Iron Phosphate
Source: Mineral
Natural mineral occurring as a brown powder of formula $Fe_3 (PO_4)_2$.

Modalities

Symptoms better for cold applications.

Symptoms worse for touch, motion and on the right side and about 4 to 6 a.m.

Constitutional Factors

Especially active for nervous, sensitive, anemic people who flush easily and may be prone to chest troubles.

Therapeutic Index:

Appetite Craving	Giddiness	Obesity
Colds	Incontinence	Otitis
Debility	Nosebleed	Shoulder Pain

23. GELSEMIUM SEMPERVIRENS

Abbreviated Name: GELSEMIUM
Common Name: Yellow Jasmine
Source: Plant

The mother tincture is prepared from the fresh root of the plant.

Modalities

Symptoms better for bending forward, open air, urinating and motion.

Symptoms worse for damp weather, before thunderstorms, during summer, excitement, dismay, smoking and about 10 to 11 a.m.

Antidotes

China; Coffea.

Constitutional Factors

Especially active for children and young people, especially sensitive women of nervous, hysterical temperament.

Therapeutic Index:

Apprehension	Fright	Sciatica
Colds	Influenza	Sunstroke
Fear	Measles	Vertigo
	Mental Exhaustion	
	Panic	

24. GRAPHITES

Common Name: Black lead
Source: Element
Prepared by Hahnemann from "the purest black lead of a fine English pencil."

Modalities

Symptoms better for wrapping up and in the dark.
Symptoms worse during and after periods and before midnight.

Antidotes

Aconite; Arsen. Alb.; Nux Vomica.

Constitutional Factors

Especially active for fat, flabby people with an extremely cautious nature. They may have pale, unhealthy skin, are subject to flatulence and constipation and susceptible to cold. Women have late menstruation, breasts are large and hard and fridigity is frequent. They are fidgety, sometimes despondent, timid and indecisive.

Therapeutic Index:

Constipation	Insomnia	Sexual Problems
Dandruff	Itching	Stings
Deafness	Menopause	Styes
Eczema	Nail Problems	Tinnitus
Feet Discomfort	Obesity	Warts
	Psoriasis	

25. HAMAMELIS VIRGINIANA

Abbreviated Name: HAMAMELIS
Common Name: Witch Hazel
Source: Plant
This remedy was proven by Dr. Constantine Hering in the United States.

The mother tincture is prepared from the root of the plant when the leaves are falling.

Modalities

Symptoms better for being outdoors.

Symptoms worse for warm, damp air, from touch and during the day.

Antidotes

None listed.

Constitutional Factors

Especially active for people who demand respect and are liable to suffer from varicose veins or hemorrhage.

Therapeutic Index:

Anal Disorders	Hemorrhoids	Ulcers
Bruises	Nosebleed	Varicose Veins
	Swollen Ankles	

26. HEPAR SULFURIS

Abbreviated Name: HEPAR SULF.
Common Name: Calcium Sulfide
Source: Mineral
One of the earliest remedies introduced by Hahnemann, which he prepared by burning equal parts of the middle layer of oyster shells (calcium carbonate) with flowers of sulfur at high temperature.

Yellowish white powder of formula CaS (calcium sulfide).

Modalities

Symptoms better for damp weather, warmth (particularly round the head) and after eating.

Symptoms worse for dry, cold weather (during winter), drafts, touch and after eating.

Antidotes

Acidum Acet.; Arsen. Alb.; Chamomilla; Silica.

Constitutional Factors

Especially active for people with light hair and complexion, unsociable, slow moving, elderly and subject to glandular swellings.

Therapeutic Index:

Abscesses	Burns	Mouth Ulcers
Acne	Carbuncles	Urticaria
Anger	Colds	Whitlows
Appetite Craving	Croup	Wounds
	Laryngitis	
	Lips	

27. HYDRASTIS CANADENSIS

Abbreviated Name: HYDRASTIS
Common Name: Golden Seal
Source: Plant

Modalities

Symptoms better for cold air.
Symptoms worse for physical exertion.

Antidote

Sulfur.

Constitutional Factors

Especially active in older, debilitated people who easily tire and who may suffer from catarrh and depression.

Therapeutic Index:

Constipation	Sore Throat	Tongue Disorders
Deafness	Tinnitus	

28. HYPERICUM PERFORATUM

Abbreviated Name: HYPERICUM
Common Name: St. John's Wort

Source: Plant

The mother tincture is prepared from the whole plant.

Modalities

Symptoms better for bending head backward.

Symptoms worse for cold, damp, closed rooms, exposure, touch and about 3 to 4 a.m.

Antidotes

Arsen Alb.; Chamomilla; Sulfur.

Constitutional Factors

Especially active for people who suffer from nervous depression, particularly after wounds or operations.

Therapeutic Index:

Anal Disorders	Concussion	Trauma
Bites	Mouth Ulcers	Wounds (crushed
Bruises	Sexual Problems	fingers and toes
Coccyx Pain	Toothache	and punctures)

29. IGNATIA AMARA

Abbreviated Name: IGNATIA

Common Name: St. Ignatius' Bean

Source: Plant

Introduced by Hahnemann in his *Fragmenta di Viribus Medicamentorum*, published in 1805.

The mother tincture is prepared from the seeds of the plant.

Modalities

Symptoms better while eating, for warmth, hard pressure, walking, change of position.

Symptoms worse in the morning, after meals, in open air, after smoking, strong odors and grief.

Antidotes

Pulsatilla; Chamomilla; Cocculus; Arnica: Acid Acet.

Constitutional Factors

Especially active for people who are over-sensitive in mind and body, with a nervous temperament. Dark-haired women of a sensitive, emotional, nervous disposition, mild, tearful, perceptive, easily excited, contradictory and rapid in execution and dislike tobacco. (Contrast with Pulsatilla).

Therapeutic Index:

Anal Disorders	Emotional Problems	Loss of Appetite
Bereavement	Fainting	Menopause
Croup	Fear	Numbness
Depression	Hoarseness	Sexual Problems
Distended Abdomen	Hypochondria	Travel Sickness
	Jet Lag	

30. IPECACUANHA

Common Name: Ipecac
Source: Plant
The mother tincture is prepared from the entire dried root of the plant.

Modalities

Symptoms worse for moist, warm wind, slightest motion, lying down, in winter and about 11 a.m.

Antidotes

China; Nux Vom.; Tabacam.

Constitutional Factors

Especially active for overweight children and adults, prone to nausea and colds.

Therapeutic Index:

Asthma	Nausea	Vomiting
Bronchitis	Saliva, Excess	Whooping Cough
	Travel Sickness	

31. KALI BICHROMICUM

Abbreviated Name: KALI BICH.
Common Name: Bichromate of Potash
Source: Mineral
Bright orange-red crystals of formula $K_2Cr_2O_7$

Modalities

Symptoms better for cold weather.
Symptoms worse for hot, summer weather, undressing and about 2 to 3 a.m.

Antidotes

Arsen Alb.; Lachesis; Pulsatilla.

Constitutional Factors

Especially active for pale, overweight people, particularly children, prone to catarrh with general weakness.

Therapeutic Index:

Bone Pains	Cough	Giddiness
Bronchitis	Croup	Headache
Catarrh	Dyspepsia	Laryngitis
Concussion	Excitement	Measles

32. KALI PHOSPHORICUM

Abbreviated Name: KALI PHOS.
Common Name: Potassium Phosphate
Source: Mineral
White powder of formula K_3PO_4.

Modalities

Symptoms better for warmth, rest or gentle movement and after meals.

Symptoms worse for physical exertion, noise, worry, excitement, eating and cold.

Constitutional Factors

Especially active for shy people with poor memory, liable to be nervous, become overexcited, particularly young people.

Therapeutic Index:

Bites	Boils	Excitement
Blisters	Change of Life	Giddiness

33. LACHESIS MUTUS

Abbreviated Name: LACHESIS
Common Name: Bushmaster Snake Venom
Source: Animal
Originally proved by Dr. Constantine Hering, from the venom of snake, during his travels in South America.

Modalities

Symptoms better for warm applications.

Symptoms worse after sleep, pressure, constriction, in the spring and for hot drinks and acid food, on left side moving to right.

Antidotes

Arsen Alb.; Acidum Nit.; Belladonna; Chamomilla; Cocules; Carbo Veg.; Coffea; Alum.

Constitutional Factors

Especially active for people of a melancholic disposition, with dark complexions. Women with freckles and red hair. Jealousy and suspicion dominate, talkative.

Therapeutic Index:

Abdominal Pain	Hysteria	Sore Throat
Alcoholism	Pains	Tinnitus

34. LEDUM PALUSTRE

Abbreviated Name: LEDUM
Common Name: Wild Rosemary
Source: Plant
Introduced by Hahnemann, the mother tincture is prepared from the whole fresh plant.

Modalities

Symptoms better for cold.
Symptoms worse from heat in bed and at night.

Antidotes

Camphor.

Constitutional Factors

Especially active for robust, red-faced people who may be discontented at times. They often feel cold or chilly.

Therapeutic Index:

Arthritis	Muscle Pains	Rheumatic Conditions
Gout	Puncture Wounds	Wounds
	Respiratory Conditions	

35. LYCOPODIUM CLAVATUM

Abbreviated Name: LYCOPODIUM
Common Name: Club Moss
Source: Plant
Originally proved by Hahnemann et al. The mother tincture is prepared from the crushed spores of the plant.

Modalities

Symptoms better for warm food and drinks, motion, getting cold by removing clothes and after midnight.

Symptoms worse for warm rooms, in bed and usually between 4 and 8 p.m.

Antidotes

Aconite; Causticum; Chamomilla; Graphites; Pulsatilla.

Constitutional Factors

Especially active for tall, thin, intellectual people who are physically weak and lack stamina, with sallow complexion and possibly freckles. They are conscientious, cautious and liable to loss of self-confidence, apprehensive, but can be headstrong.

Therapeutic Index:

Abdominal pains	Flatulence	Sexual Problems
Acidity	Headache	Sprains
Appetite Craving	Hiccough	Swelling
Apprehension	Hypocondria	Tongue Disorders
Deafness	Pains	Tonsillitis
Depression	Premenstrual Syndrome	Urticaria
Feet Discomfort	Sciatica	Yawning

36. MAGNESIA PHOSPHORICUM

Abbreviated Name: MAG. PHOS.
Common Name: Magnesium Phosphate
Source: Mineral
White powder of formula $Mg_3(PO_4)_2$

Modalities

Symptoms better for warmth, pressure, friction and bending double.

Symptoms worse for cold air, cold bathing, motion, touch, at night and on right side.

Antidotes

Belladonna; Gelsemium; Lachesis.

Constitutional Factors

Especially active for very thin people with a dark complexion. They may be tired or exhausted, dislike mental effort and be very nervous.

Therapeutic Index:

Belching	Neuralgia	Toothache
Nettle Rash	Pains	

37. MERCURIUS VIVUS

Abbreviated Name: MERC. VIV.
Common Name: Mercury
Source: Element
Quicksilver. Originally proved by Hahnemann in soluble form (Merc. Sol).

Modalities

No listed ameliorations.

Symptoms worse for wet, damp weather, perspiring, warm rooms, lying on right side and at night.

Antidotes

Belladonna; Bryonia; Carbo Veg.; Cuprum Met.; Aceticum Nit; Kali Bich.; Lachesis; Nux Vomica; Phytolacca; Staphysagria; Spigelia; Sulfur; Stramonium; Sepia; Hepar Sulf.

Constitutional Factors

Especially active for fair-haired people with lax skin and muscles, who perspire easily.

Therapeutic Index:

Bad Breath	Candida Infection	Sore Throat
Bronchitis	Influenza	Tongue Disorders
Colds	Pyorrhea	Toothache
	Rheumatism	

38. NATRUM MURIATICUM

Abbreviated Name: NATRUM MUR.
Common Name: Sodium Chloride (Common Salt)
Source: Mineral
Common salt of formula NaCl from natural rock salt.

Modalities

Symptoms better for the open air, cold bathing, pressure on back and lying on right side.

Symptoms worse for mental exertion, noise, music, lying down, heat, talking, by the seashore and between 10 and 11 a.m.

Antidotes

Arsen Alb.; Phosphorus; Sepia; Nux Vomica.

Constitutional Factors

Especially active for anemic people through loss of body fluids or mental affections, women with profuse periods, subject to weariness and colds.

Therapeutic Index:

Blisters	Herpes	Menstrual Disorders
Catarrh	Hypochondria	Mental Exhaustion
Colds	Lips	Premenstrual Syndrome

39. NUX VOMICA

Abbreviated name: NUX VOM.
Common Name: Poison Nut
Source: Plant
Introduced by Hahnemann in his book *Fragmenta di Viribus Medicamentorum* in 1805.

The mother tincture is prepared from the dried seeds of the berries of the tree.

Modalities

Symptoms better for resting, wet, damp weather, strong pressure and in the evening.

Symptoms worse for mental exertion, overeating, touch, noise, stimulants, alcohol, dry weather, cold air and between 3 and 4 a.m.

Constitutional Factors

Especially active for thin, active, irritable, nervous, hyperactive, dark-haired people. Typically, the overworked executive who gets inadequate exercise and calms himself or herself with coffee, alcohol or by smoking. Prone to indigestion and biliousness or hemorrhoids and readily chilled.

Therapeutic Index:

Abdominal Pains	Bilious Attack	Loss of Appetite
Acidity	Breath, Bad	Lumbago
Acne Rosacea	Constipation	Jet Lag
Aggressiveness	Depression	Muscular Pain
Alcoholism	Diarrhea	Nosebleed
Anal Disorders	Dyspepsia	Sexual Problems
Asthma	Headache	Weakness
	Hiccough	
	Jaundice	

40. PHOSPHORUS

Common Name: Phosphorus
Source: Mineral
Red, allotropic form of phosphorus from natural phosphate rock.

Modalities

Symptoms better for cold food, in the dark, open air, sleep, rubbing and lying on the right side.

Symptoms worse for touch, during thunderstorms or change of weather, ascending stairs, lying on left or affected side and before midnight.

Antidotes

Coffea; Nux Vomica; Sepia; Calc. Carb.

Constitutional Factors

Especially active for tall, fair or red-haired brainy people with pale skin, delicate eyelashes. Over-sensitive to environment—light, sound, odors, touch. Experience sudden symptoms. Young people growing fast and old people, possibly with diarrhea in the morning.

Therapeutic Index:

Anal Disorders	Chestiness	Laryngitis
Belching	Cough	Nosebleed
Bone Pains	Hoarseness	Perspiration
Bronchitis	Jaundice	Vomiting

41. PHYTOLACCA DECANDRA

Abbreviated Name: PHYTOLACCA
Common Name: Poke Weed
Source: Plant
The mother tincture is prepared from the whole plant, including the berries.

Modalities

Symptoms better for warmth, rest, dry weather.

Symptoms worse for rain, damp, cold weather, night air, electric charges.

Antidotes

Belladonna; Mezereum.

Constitutional Factors

Especially active for thin, rheumatic people who tire easily and who lose weight.

Therapeutic Index:

Boils   Premenstrual Syndrome   Tonsillitis
Neuralgia   Sore Throat

42. PULSATILLA NIGRICANS

Abbreviated Name: PULSATILLA
Common Name: Windflower
Source: Plant
Introduced by Hahnemann in his book *Fragmenta di Viribus Medicamentorum* in 1805. Sometimes called the "Sunset Remedy." The mother tincture is prepared from the whole, fresh flowering plant in spring or fall.

Modalities

Symptoms better for open air, cold air or cool room, motion, cold food and drinks, cold applications.

Symptoms worse for warm rooms, after eating, rich or indigestible food, heat, warm applications, lying down on left or painless side at about 4 p.m.

Antidotes

Coffea; Chamomilla; Ignatia; Nux Vomica; Stannum Met.

Constitutional Factors

Chief guide to the choice of this remedy.

Females, particularly young girls with blonde or sandy hair, blue eyes and pale, delicate complexion. She is romantic, emotional, easily moved to laughter and tears, even on a slight reprimand. Affectionate, mild and gentle, fearful, friendly and shy. She is indecisive, yielding, with changeable moods and dislikes cold, although she likes cool places. She often lies with her hands above her head.

Therapeutic Index:

Abdominal Pain   Conjunctivitis   Mumps
Acne   Deafness   Nausea
Acute Bronchitis   Excitement   Premenstrual Syndrome
Arthritis   Gout   Sexual Problems
Catarrh   Headache   Sinus Obstruction
Chicken Pox   Incontinence   Toothache
Chilblains   Joint Pain   Urticaria
Colds   Measles   Weakness

43. RHUS TOXICODENDRON

Abbreviated Name: RHUS TOX.
Common Name: Poison Ivy
Source: Plant
The mother tincture is prepared from the dark green leaves freshly gathered before flowering and after sunset.

Modalities

Symptoms better for warm, dry weather, motion, walking, change of position, rubbing, movements of affected parts, stretching limbs.

Symptoms worse for cold, before storms, during sleep, wet weather, lying on back on right side and when perspiring, in the Fall, about 7 p.m. and at night.

Antidotes

Aconite; Belladonna; Bryonia; Camphor; Coffea; Croton Tig.; Graphites; Lachesis; Sulfur; Sepia.

Constitutional Factors

Especially active for people of rheumatic diathesis affected by getting wet or overheated. They are restless, prone to depression, apprehensive at night and prefer to be alone.

Therapeutic Index:

Acne Rosacea	Conjunctivitis	Rheumatism
Backache	Herpes	Sprains
Bursitis	Joint Pain	Sunburn
Chicken Pox	Ligament Pain	Tongue Disorders
	Lumbago	
	Pains	

44. RUTA GRAVEOLENS

Abbreviated Name: RUTA GRAV.
Common Name: Bitterwort
Source: Plant
A medicinal herb known to early civilizations.

Modalities

No ameliorations listed.

Symptoms are worse for lying down, cold, wet weather and on initial movement after resting.

Antidotes

Camphor.

Constitutional Factors

Especially active for anxious people, dissatisfied with self and others, with tendency to weakness and despair.

Therapeutic Index:

Bone Pains	Fractures	Trauma
Bruises	Rheumatism	Weakness
	Sprains	

5. SEPIA OFFICINALIS

Abbreviated Name: SEPIA
Common Name: Ink of Cuttlefish
Source: Animal
Brown, inky juice exuded from sac of the cuttlefish on the approach of a predator.

Modalities

Symptoms better for pressure, warm bed, hot applications, strenuous exercise, drawing up limbs, cold bathing and after sleep.

Symptoms worse for damp, cold air, before thunderstorms, evening, on left side and strenuous exercise (also ameliorate).

Antidotes

Aconite; Antimonium Crud.; Sulfur; Antimonium Tart.

Constitutional Factors

Especially active for thin, dark-haired persons below average height, especially *women* of mild disposition. They may be indolent and fearful and easily depressed with a dislike of fatty and starchy foods.

Therapeutic Index:

Appetite Craving	Hair Loss	Nail Problems
Change of Life	Herpes	Premenstrual Syndrome
Dandruff	Incontinence	Swelling
	Menopause	

46. SILICA

Common Name: Pure Flint
Source: Mineral

White powder of transparent crystals of formula SiO_2.

Modalities

Symptoms better for warmth, especially wrapping up head, in summer.

Symptoms worse for cold, during periods, uncovering the head, lying down, and in the evening and in winter.

Antidotes

Acidum Fluor; Camphor; Hepar Sulf.

Constitutional Factors

Especially active for people with fine, dry skin and pale complexion, nervous, irritable, weakly with lax muscles. Oversensitive, physically and mentally. Scrofulous children with large heads and distended abdomen.

Therapeutic Index:

Abscesses	Carbuncles	Headache
Acne	Coccyx Pain	Loss of Appetite
Appetite Craving	Constipation	Nail Problems
Boils	Deafness	Perspiration
Bone Pains	Debility	Pyorrhea
Bunions	Distended Abdomen	Ulcers
	Feet Discomfort	
	Hay Fever	

47. SULFUR

Common Name: Sulfur
Source: Mineral (Element)
Introduced by Hahnemann, although known as a medicament in early civilizations.

Modalities

Symptoms better for dry, warm weather, and lying on the right side.

Symptoms worse for rest or standing, in warm bed, from alcohol, washing, changeable weather, in the morning about 11 a.m.

Antidotes

Aconite; Camphor; Chamomilla; China; Causticum; Nux Vomica; Merc. Sol.

Constitutional Factors

Especially active for people with dry, hard skin and red orifices. People of nervous temperament, quick-tempered, quick-motioned, dyspeptic, inclined to be selfish, perspire easily with body odor. Independent, thinking people who may have a stoop which gives them the appearance of being older.

Therapeutic Index:

Adenoids	Candida Infection	Itching
Alcoholism	Dandruff	Perspiration
Anal Disorders	Diarrhea	Psoriasis
Appetite	Eczema	Rheumatism
Belching	Emotional Problems	Ringworm
Body Odor	Feet Discomfort	Sexual Problems
Bronchitis	Insomnia	Tinnitus

48. SYMPHYTUM OFFICINALIS

Abbreviated Name: SYMPHYTUM
Common Name: Comfrey
Source: Plant
The mother tincture is prepared from the root of the plant.

Modalities

None listed.

Antidotes

Aconite; Merc. Viv.; Sabadilla; Camphor; Hepar Sulf.

Constitutional Factors

Of little significance.

Therapeutic Index:

Bruises	Eye Injury	Trauma
	Fractures	

49. THUJA OCCIDENTALIS

Abbreviated Name: THUJA
Common Name: Tree of Life
Source: Plant
The mother tincture is prepared from the fresh, green branches.

Modalities

Symptoms better for drawing up a limb and on left side.
Symptoms worse for heat of bed, cold, damp, fatty foods,

coffee, after vaccination, about 3 a.m. and 3 p.m. and in the Fall.

Antidotes

Camphor; Cocculus; Chamomilla; Merc. Sol.; Pulsatilla; Sulfur; Staphysagria; Sabina (warts).

Constitutional Factors

Especially active for dark, dry-haired people with dark complexion.

Therapeutic Index:

Apprehension	Joint Pain	Warts
Distended Abdomen	Nail Problems	

50. URTICA URENS

Common Name: Stinging Nettle
Source: Plant
The mother tincture is prepared from the fresh, flowering plant.

Modalities

Symptoms better for warm, dry air.
Symptoms worse for cold, contact with water, coal, moist air and touch.

Antidotes

None listed.

Constitutional Factors

Especially active for plump people with dark hair and dark complexion, unhealthy skin. May feel fragile. Ill effects from vaccinations or eating shellfish.

Therapeutic Index:

Burns	Insomnia	Sunburn
Gout	Itching	Urticaria
	Stings	

APPENDICES

1. NOSODES (INCLUDING BOWEL NOSODES)

Acne Bacillus
Actinomyces
Amoeba
Anaphylactic Lung
Anthracinum
Anti-Catarrh Vaccine
Anti-Coli Baccilaire
Arteriosclerosis
Ascarides

Bacillinum
Bacillus Dispar
Bacillus Dysenterii
Bacillus No. 10 (Paterson)
Bacillus Pyogenes
Bacillus Subtilus
Bacillus Tetani (Tetanus)
Bacillus Welchii
Bordetella Pertussis
Bothrocephalus
Botulinum
Brucella Abortus
Brucella Melitensis
Brucellos Abortus
Bulbaparalysis

Calc Renalis
Candida Alba (ex bird)
Candida Albicans (Monilia Albicans)
Carcinoma
Caroinosin
Cat Enteritis
Cat Leukaemia
Cataract
Cataractin
Catarrh Vaccine
Chlamydia

Chlamydia Trach.
Coccal Co.
Corynebacterium Anaerobe
Cytomegalo Virus

Dandruff
Deforman
Diphtherinum
Disseminated Sclerosis (Sclerosin)
Distemperinum
Diverticulosis
Dysenteria

E. Coli
Encephalitis
Entamoeba Coli
Entamoeba Hist.
Enterococcinum
Enteritis
Equine Melanoma
Erysipelas

Faecalis (Bach)
Filaria
Folliculinum
Friedlander (Bacillus F)

Gaertner (Bach)
Glandular Fever

Haemophilus Influenziae
Hepatitis Nosode
Herpes Mammalitis
Herpes Progenitalis
Herpes Simplex
Herpes Simplex Virus B
Herpes Zoster
H.E. Coli Type E57

Hippozaeninum (Mallein)
Hodgkins Disease
Husk Nosode
Hydrophobinum (Lyssin)
Infectious Keratitis
Influenza A Chile 1983
Influenza A England
Influenza A Mississipi
　1985
Influenza B Ann Arbor
　1986
Influenza B Hong Kong
Influenza B/HK, A/Texas,
　A/USSR
Influenza 1984 (W.H.O.)
Influenzinum (Bangkok,
　Singapore, Brazil)
Influezinum (Influenza
　Bach. Poly'flu)

K. Pneumonia
Kieferostitis Nosode
Klebsiella

Legionella
Leptospirosis
Leuco-Encaphalitis
Leukemia (Lymphoblastic)
Leukemia (Myeloblastic)
Lymphosarcoma

Malandrinum
Malaria Officinalis
Malaria Tropical
Mastitis
Measles Vaccine
Medorrhinum
Melanoma Sarcomium
Meningeoma Nosode
Micrococcus Catarrhalis
Morbillinum
Morgan (Bach)
Morgan Gaertner
Morgan Pure
Mucobacter
Mucobacter (Catarrh
　Vaccine)
Multiple Sclerosis
Mutabile
Mucoplasma Pneumonia
Myxomatosis

Nasal Cararrh
Nasal Polyp

Orf Nosode
Osteomyelitis

Paratyphoid A
Paratyphoid B
Parkinsons
Parotidinum
Parvo Virus
Penicillin Notatum
Pertinum (Yersin)
Pertussin
Pertussis Vaccine
Plaque (dental)
Pneumococcus
Polio Nosode (Salk
　Vaccine)
Polybowel Co.
Polyvalent (Bach)
Polyvalent Catarrh
　Vaccine
Proteus (Bach)
Pseudomonas (ex cancine)
Psittacosis
Psoriasis
Psorinum
Pyelonephritis
Pyrogenium (Sepsin)

Rabies
Rheumatoid Arthritic
　Nosode Knee
Rheumatoid O.A.N.
Rous Sarcoma
Rubella

Salmonella
Scarlatinum
Scirrhinum
Septioaemin
Spengler
Staphylococcus
　Abdominalis
Staphylococcus Albus
Staphylococcus Aureus
Staphylococcus Coagula-
　tion Positive
Streptococcus
Streptococcus
　Haemolvticus Aurues
Streptococcus Pneumoniae
　(Tl)
Streptococcus
　Rheumaticus

Streptococcus Viridans
Cardiacus
Streptococcus Virus 'Flu.
Sycotic Co.
Syphlilinum (Leuticum,
Luesinum,
Brossulinum)
Tetanus Antitoxin
Tetanus Toxin
Tonsillinum
Toxoplasmosis
Trichinosis
Trichomonas
Triple Vaccine
Tuberculinum Aviare
Tuberculinum Bovinum
Tuberculinum Kent
Tuberculinum Klebs

Tuberculinum Koch (T.K.)
Tuberculinum Koch
Exotoxin
Tuberculinum (Nebel)
Tuberculinum Residuum
Tuberculinum Rosen
Tuberculinum Test
Typhinum
Typhoidinum
Toxoplasma (equine)

Vaccininum
Vaccinosis
Varicella
Variolinum
Vincent's Angina
Virus Pneumonia

Yellow Fever

2. ALLERGENS

Alder
Allspice
Almonds
Alternaria
Alternaria
Tenuis
American
Cheese
American Elm
American
Hazelnut
Animal
Glycerine
Anise Seed
Apple
Apricot
Arizona Cypress
Artichoke
Ash
Asparagus
Aspergillus
Aspergillus
Fumigatus
Aspergillus
Glaucus
Aspergillus
Niger
Aspergillus
Terreus
Avocado

Bahia
Baker's Yeast
Bamboo
Banana
Barley
Barley Smut
Basil
Bay Leaves
Beef
Beer
Bermuda Grass
Bermuda Grass
Smut
Birch
Black Pepper
Black Willow
Blackberry
Blackeyed Pea
Blue Dye
Blueberry
Botrytis
Cinereas
Boysenberry
Brandy
Brewer's Yeast
Broccoli
Brussels Sprouts
Buckwheat
Butter
Cabbage

Calf's Liver
Candida
(Monilla Alb.)
Caraway Seed
Carrot
Cashew Nut
Cat's Hair
Cauliflower
Celery
Cement
Cephalasporium
Cephalothecium
Chaetomium
Globosum
Cheddar Cheese
Cheese
Cherry
Chicken
Chinese Elm
Chlorine
Chocolate
Cladosporium
Clam
Cloves
Coconut
Codfish
Coffee
Common
Sagebrush
Concord Grape

Concrete
Corn
Corn Smut
Cottage Cheese
Cotton
Cottonseed
Cottonwood
Crab
Cucumber
Cultivated Corn
Curry Powder
Dacron
Date Palm
Dementia
Dill Seed
Dog Hair
Egg
Egg Plant
English Plantain
Epicoccum Spp.
Epidermophyton
Flocconum
European Olive
Fat (Edible)
Feathers
Fig
Firebush
Flaxseed
Flea

Flounder
Fluoride
Fusarium
  Oxysporum
Fusarium Spp.
Garlic
Geotrichum
  Candidum
Getreidepollen
Gigartina
  Mammil
Gigartina
  Seaweed
Gin
Ginger
Gliocladium
  Spp.
Gluten
Grain Dust
Grain Sorghum
Grape (Raisin)
Grapefruit
Grass, Canary
Grass, Early
Grass, Grama
  Blue
Grass, Johnson
Grass, Late
Grass, Orchard
Grass, Pollen
  (All varieties)
Grass, Quack
Grass, Redtop
Grass, Rye
Grass, Salt
Grass, Timothy
Grass, Western
  June
Grass, Western
  Wheat
Greasewood
Green Olive
Hackberry
Haddock
Halibut
Ham
Hay Dust
Heather Honey
Helminthospo-
  rium Spp.
Hemlock

Hickory
Histamine
Histaminum
Hydro-
  chloricum
Honey
Hops
Hormodendrum
Horse Hair
Horseradish
House Dust
House Dust
  Mite
Hydrocarbons
Karaya Gum
Lamb's Quarter
Lemon
Lettuce
Lima Bean
Lime
Malt
Maple
Margarine
Meadow Fescue
Mesquite
Microsporum
  Audouini
Microsporum
  Canis
Milk
Mold Mix
Monilia
Monosodium
  Glutamate
Monotospora
Mosquito
Mountain
  Cedar
Mucor Mecedo
Mucor
  Plumbeus
Mucor
  Racemosus
Mustard
Mycogone Spp.
Navy Bean
Neurospora
  Sitophila
Newsprint
Nigrospora Spp.

Nutmeg
Oak
Oak Smut
Oats
Okra
Onion
Orange
Oregano
Papaya
Paprika
Parsley
Parsnip
Peach
Peanut
Pear
Peas
Pecan
Pennicillium
  Chrysogenium
Pennicillium
  Notatum
Pennicillium
  Rubrum
Pepper, Green
Phenol
Pigweed
Pine
Pineapple
Pinto Beans
Plant Fat
Plasma, Horse
Plum
Pollatin
Pollen, Mixed
  (South Africa)
Pollen, Pine
  Tree
Poppy Seed
Pork
Potato
Privet
Provera
Pullularia
  Pullulans
Pumpkin
Pussy Willow
Radish
Ragweed
Red Dye
Red Mulberry

Rhizopus
  Nigrocans
Rhodotorula
Rhoma
  Destructiva
Rhubarb
Rice
Ripe Olive
Rough
  Marshelder
Rubber
Russian Thistle
Rye
Rye Grass
Saccharin
Safflower Seed
  Oil
Sage
Sagebrush
  Dragon
Salmon
Sawdust
Scallops
Scopulariopsis
Sea Salt
Sesame Seeds
Sodium Nitrate
Sorghum Smut
Sorrel
Soybean
Spinach
Spondylocl
  Atrovirens
Sporotrichum
  Pruinosum
Squash
Stemphylium
Stinging Insects
  (mix)
Strawberry
String Bean
Sugar Beet
Sugar Cane
Sugar Deposits
Sweet Potato
Sweet Vernal
Sycamore
Sycamore Alba.
Tea
Terpene
Thyme

Tobacco
Tomato, Raw
Trichoderma Spp.
Trichophyton Mentagrophytes
Trichophyton Rubrum
Trichophyton Tonsurans

Tuna
Turkey
Turnip
Vanilla
Veg. Glycerine
Verticillium Albo-Atrum
Vinegar (Apple Cider)
Vinegar (Malt)

Vinegar (Wine)
Walnut
Water Hemp
Wheat (Cultivated)
Wheat (Whole)
Wheat Manna
Wheat Smut
Wheat Stem Rust

Whisky
White Poplar
White Rose Oil
Whole Cherry
Wine
Wingscale
Wooley Ragweed
Yeast
Yellow Dye

3. ORGANOTHERAPY PREPARATIONS (SARCODES)

Acoustic Nerve
Adrenal Cortex
Adrenal Gland
Adrenal Medulla
Anal Mucosa
Anterior Lobe Pituitary
Aorta
Appendix
Aqueous Vitreous
Atlas
Auricle
Auriculoventricular Wall

Bile
Billary Canal
Bladder
Blood
Blood Plasma
Bone Marrow
Bone of Ear
Brachial Plexus
Brain
Bronchus
Buccale Mucosa
Bulbinum

Caecum
Callosum
Capillary Tissue
Cardia of Stomach
Carotid Artery
Carotid Plexus
Cartilage
Celiac Plexus
Cerebellum
Cerebral Artery
Cerebral Cortex

Cerebral Cortex and Hypothal
Cerebrinum
Cervical Discus
Cervical Medulla
Cervical Vertebra
Choroid
Cillary Zone
Circumvolupic of Hippocampus
Coccyx
Coccyx Femoral Cartilage
Colon Mucosa
Conjuctiva
Connecting Cartilage
Connective Tissue
Coronary Artery
Coronary Vein
Cornea
Crystalline Lens
Cubital Nerve
Cystis Canal

Deferns Canal
Diaphragm
Diencephalon
Dorsal Medulla
Dorsal Vertebra
Duodenum

Eardrum
Encephalon
Endocardium
Epididymis
Epiphysis
Erectile Tissue
Esophagus
Eustachium

Eye
Eye Muscle

Facial Tissue
Fallopian Tube
Fatty Tissue
Femoral Artery
Fibrin
Flat Bone
Frontal Lobe

Gall Bladder
Gastric Mucosa
Glossopharyngeal Nerve
Grey Substance (Nerve)
Gum Mucosa

Hair Bulb
Heart
Hematopoietic Tissue
Hemorrhoidal Vein
Hepatic Canal
Hypogastric Plexus
Hypothalamus

Inner Ear
Intestine Mucosa

Jejunum
Joints Capsule
Joints of Ankle
Joints of Elbow
Joints of Hip
Joints of Knee
Joints of Shoulder

Kidney
Kidney Medulla
Knee Meniscus

Labyrinth of Ear
Lacrymal Fluid
Large Intestine
Larynx
Left Colon
Left Ventricle
Ligament
Ligament Art. Elbow
Ligament Art. Hip
Ligament Art. Knee
Ligament Art.
  Shoulder
Liquor Cerebro
  Spinalis
Liver
Long Bone
Lumbar Discus
Lumbar Medulla
Lumbar Vertebrae
Lung
Lutein
Lymph Node
Lymphatic Vessels

Mammary Gland
Median Nerve
Medulla
Mesencephalon
Middle Ear
Mitral Valve
Motor Nerve
Myocardium

Nasal Mucosa
Neck of Bladder
Neck of Womb
Nerve
Nonstriated Muscle

Occipital Lobe
Occipital Nerve
Oddi's Sphincter
Odontoid Vertebrae

Olfactory Lobe
Olfactory Nerve
Opthalmic Artery
Optic Chiasm
Optic Nerve
Ovary

Pancreas
Pancreatic Canal
Parasympathetic
  Nerve
Parathyroid
Parietallobe
Partoid
Pelvic Colon
Pericardium
Periosteum
Peritoneum
Pharnyx
Pituitary Gland
Placenta
Pleura
Post Pituitary
Prostate
Pulmonary Artery
Pylorus Mucosa
Quadrigeminal Bodies,
  Brain
Radial Nerve
Rectosigmoid Mucosa
Rectum
Red Corpuscle
Renal Cortex
Retina
Rhinenciphalus
Rhinophargeal Mucosa
Right Colon
Right Ventricule

Sacral Medulla
Sacral Piexus
Sacral Vertebrae

Salivary Gland
Sciatic Nerve
Seminal Vescicle
Serum
Short Bone
Sinus Mucosa
Small Intestine
Spleen
Spongy Tissue
Stomach
Striated Muscle
Sympathetic Nerve
Synovium

Temporal Lobe
Tendon
Testicle
Thalamus
Thoracic Discus
Thymus
Thyroid
Tongue
Tonsil
Tooth
Trachea
Transverse Colon
Trigeminal Nerve
True Skin

Ureter
Urethra
Uterus

Vaginal Mucosa
Vein
Vena Cava Inferior
Vena Sphena
Ventricule
Vertebrae
Vertebral Discus
Vertebral Ligament
Vesicae
Vitreum
Vulva

4. HOMEOPATHIC ORGANIZATIONS IN THE UNITED STATES

National Organizations

California, Alhambra

American Foundation for Homeopathy (AFH). Est. 1924.
1508 Garfield, Alhambra, CA 91801.

This is a non-profit organization to promote homeopathy in the United States. It continues today primarily as a fund-raising and educational entity.

California, Orinda

California State Homeopathic Medical Society. Est. 1877.
10 Hillcrest Drive, Orinda, CA 94563.
This is a professional, non-profit organization to promote homeopathy in the Western States.

District of Columbia

American Board of Homeotherapeutics (ABHT). Est. 1960.
1500 Massachusetts Avenue, N.W., Washington, D.C. 20005.
This is the certifying homeopathic specialty board for licensed U.S. physicians and osteopaths who meet its prerequisites and pass its examinations.

American Institute of Homeopathy (AIH). Est. 1844.
1500 Massachusetts Avenue, N.W., Washington, D.C. 20005.
The oldest national medical professional organization in the United States, the AIH was established to improve homeopathic therapeutics and education, to maintain standards of homeopathic practice, to disseminate homeopathic medical knowledge, and to promote public acceptance of homeopathy.

National Center for Homeopathy (NCH). Est. 1974.
1500 Massachusetts Avenue, N.W., Washington, D.C. 20005; tel., 202-223-6182.
A non-profit public membership organization, the NCH promotes homeopathy in the United States by education, publications, research and membership services. It is the spiritual descendant of the American Foundation for Homeopathy.

Ohio

Ohio State Homeopathic Medical Society. Est. 1864.
5148 S. State Road, Route 202, Tipp City, OH 45317.
A professional medical society, it was established for the promotion, advancement and safeguarding of homeopathic medicine in Ohio.

Pennsylvania, Lancaster

Homeopathic Medical Society of the State of Pennsylvania. Est. 1866.
P.O. Box 153, Lancaster, PA 17604.
This society was formed to organize and support the homeopathic medical profession in Pennsylvania.

Pennsylvania, Norwood

Homeopathic Pharmacopoeia Convention of the United States. Est. 1980.
126 W. Garfield, Avenue, Box 174, Norwood, PA 19074.
This is a non-profit organization charged with the preparation and the publication of the *Homeopathic Pharmacopoeia of the United States*.

Women's Homeopathic League, Inc.
126 W. Garfield Avenue, Norwood, PA 19074.

Virginia, Fairfax

Southern Homeopathic Medical Association. Est. 1885.
10418 Whitehead St., Fairfax, VA 22030. Tel., 703-273-5250.
The SHMA is a professional organization formed to promote homeopathic medicine, advance homeopathic education and safeguard homeopathic practice in the Southern States.

Virginia, Falls Church

American Association of Homeopathic Pharmacists. Est. 1922.
P.O. Box 2273, Falls Church, VA 22042.
This is the official organization for the American homeopathic pharmacists and for those who have established branches in the U.S.

Washington, Seattle

International Foundation for Homeopathy. Est. 1978.
2366 Eastlake Avenue, #301, Seattle, WA 98102; tel., 206-324-8230.
A non-profit public organization, the IFH was created to promote the highest standards of homeopathic practice and education, and to develop a public awareness of classical homeopathy.

Other Organizations

Nevada, Las Vegas

Society for Ultramolecular Medicine. Est. 1983.
3014 Rigel Avenue, Las Vegas, NV 89102; tel., 702-871-7153.
SUM was organized to fill a void created by the recent resurgence of homeopathy and acupuncture. It publishes *American Homeopathy*, a quarterly, and it also holds an annual symposium.
The Nevada Clinic.
6105 West Tropicana Avenue, Las Vegas, NV 98103; tel., 702-871-2700.

5. MANUFACTURERS OF HOMEOPATHIC MEDICINES IN THE UNITED STATES AND CANADA

California

Standard Homeopathic Company,
P.O. Box 61607, Los Angeles, CA 90061; tel., 213-321-4284.

Maryland

Washington Homeopathic Pharmacy,
4914 Del Ray Avenue, Bethesda, MD 20814; tel., 301-656-1695.

Missouri

Luyties Pharmacal Company,
4200 Laclede Avenue, St. Louis, MO 63108; tel., 800-325-8080.

Nevada

Dolisos America Inc.
3014 Rigel Avenue, Las Vegas, NV 89102; tel., 702-871-7153.

New Jersey

Humphreys Pharmacal Company,
63 Meadow Road, Rutherford, NJ 07070; tel., 201-933-7744.

New York

Weleda, Inc.,
841 South Main Street, Spring Valley, NY 10977; tel., 914-352-6145.

Pennsylvania

Boericke and Tafel, Inc.,
1011 Arch Street, Philadelphia, PA 19107; tel., 215-922-2967.

John A. Borneman and Sons (Boiron),
1208 Amosland Road, Norwood, PA 19074; tel., 215-532-2035.

Canada

Dolisos, Inc.,
1240 Rue Beaumont, #6, Mont Royal, Quebec H3P 3E5, Canada.

6. HOMEOPATHIC HOSPITALS IN THE UNITED KINGDOM

Since there are no homeopathic hospitals in the United States, the following list is provided for those American patients and professionals who wish to visit a homeopathic hospital in the United Kingdom. These hospitals conduct courses for physicians and they are also centers for homeopathic research.

Bristol

The British Homeopathic Hospital,
Cotham Road, Cotham, Bristol BS6 6JU; tel., 0272 731231.

Glasgow

The Glasgow Homeopathic Hospital,
1000 Great Western Road, Glasgow G12 0RN; tel., 041 339 0382.

Liverpool

The Liverpool Clinic-Mossley Hill Hospital,
Park Avenue, Liverpool L18 8BU; tel., 051 724 2355.

London

The Royal London Homeopathic Hospital,
Great Ormond Street, London WC1N 3HR; tel., 01 837 8833.

Tunbridge Wells

Tunbridge Wells Homeopathic Hospital,
Church Road, Tunbridge Wells, Kent; tel., 0892 42977.

7. HOMEOPATHIC ORGANIZATIONS ABROAD

England

Liverpool

North West Friends of Homeopathy. Est. 1978.
126 Olive Mount Heights, Wavertree, Liverpool L15 8LB; tel., 051 772 8348.
The major organization in northern England, which aims to relieve sickness by homeopathic medicines, educate the general public and assist in homeopathic research.

London

The British Homeopathic Association. Est. 1902.
27A Devonshire Street, London W1N 1RJ; tel., 01 935 2163.
A registered charity, its membership includes many members of the medical and allied professionals, but it is primarily an association working with and for lay people. It publishes *Homeopathy*, a quarterly.

Faculty of Homeopathy. Est. 1844 by Frederick Harvey Foster Quin.
The Royal London Homeopathic Hospital, Great Ormond Street, London WC1N 3HR; tel., 01 837 8833.
The professional body for qualified homeopathic physicians, it has powers conferred by an Act of Parliament in 1950. Graduate teaching is arranged by the faculty. It publishes *The British Homeopathic Journal*, a quarterly.

The Hahnemann Society. Est. 1958 by Dr. Alva Benjamin.
Humane Education Centre, Avenue Lodge, Bounds Green Road, London N22 4EU; tel., 01 889 1595.
The objectives of the Society are to educate the public in the principles of homeopathy and in its safety and efficacy. It also seeks to promote the study and practice of homeopathy. It publishes *Homeopathy Today*, a quarterly.

The Homeopathic Development Foundation.
19A Cavendish Square, London W1M 9AD; tel., 01-629-3204.
An information service.

The Homeopathic Trust.
Hahnemann House, 2 Powis Place at Ormond Street, London WC1N 3HT; tel., 01-837-9469.
A registered charity for the advancement of the practice and teaching of homeopathy, as well as for research.

Oxfordshire

National Association of Homeopathic Groups. Est. 1983.

11 Wingle Tye Road, Burgess Hill, West Sussex RH15 9HR.
The association was formed to coordinate the objectives of all the
homeopathic groups of Britain and to liaise with major homeopathic,
professional and governmental groups.

Middlesex

The Hahnemann College of Homeopathy. Est. 1981.
243 The Broadway, Southall, Middx., UB1 1NF; tel., 01 843 9220.
The college offers courses for homeopathic medical practitioners, paramedics as well as postgraduate courses. Classes are held at The City
University, London, from September through July.

U.K. Homeopathic Medical Association. Est. 1986.
243 The Broadway, Southall, Middx., UB1 1NF; tel., 01 843 9220.
The objectives of the association are to establish, support and encourage
the practice of homeopathic medicine; to organize lectures, seminars
and residential courses; to publish journals, newsletters, etc., in order to
promote its objectives. It publishes *Homeopathy International* three
times a year.

West Sussex

The Society of Homeopaths. Est. 1978.
47A Canada Grove, Bognor Regis, West Sussex PO21 1DW; tel., 024
386 0678.
It was established to meet the needs of competent, professional homeopaths, and it has promulgated a set of registration standards.

France

Paris

Société Médicale de Biotherapie. Est. in 1962 by Drs. O. A. Julian and
M. Tetau.
62 rue Beaubourg, 75003 Paris; tel., 010 331 4271 9616.
The Homeopathic Association of France organized its first seminars in
1975. Since its inception, it has opened sister societies throughout
France, as well as in the United States, Canada, Spain and Holland.

India

Madras

Liga Medicorum Homeopathica Internationalis (The International Homeopathic Medical League). Est. 1925 by 14 physicians from nine countries. Its registered office is in Geneva, Switzerland.
(In 1989), D.A.U. Ramakrishman, 22 Rajarathram Street, Lilpank,
Madras 60010.
Its purpose is the promotion and development of homeopathic medicine
in the world, to provide a link between qualified medical practitioners
and also between societies and persons interested in homeopathic ques-

tions. Active members are qualified in medicine, veterinary medicine, national homeopathic societies and homeopathic hospitals. Associate Members are people with homeopathic or scientific knowledge, pharmacists, medical students, odontostomatologists, chemists, physicists and technicians able to advance homeopathy. It sponsors an International Congress, which takes place at least every three years in different countries.

Switzerland

Carouge

Homeopatia Universalis. Est. in 1987 by a unification of the members of the Société Médicale de Biotherapie of France and other countries (United States, Canada, Belgium, Netherlands, Switzerland, Italy, Tunisia, Israel, Spain, Portugal and Denmark).

BP 749-1227 Carouge; tel., 41 22 43 09 78.

Its objectives are to unify homeopathic training in all countries where it is provided to constitute a common diploma from all homeopathic training organizations and to contribute to homeopathic clinical and pharmacological research. The first International Homeopathic Congress to be organized by this organization was held in Sicily in 1988.

BIBLIOGRAPHY

Boericke, William. *Materia Medica with Repertory*. New Delhi, India: B. Jain Publishers Ltd., ND.

Borland, Douglas, M.D. *Homeopathy in Practice*. New Canaan, CT: Keats Publishing, Inc., 1982.

Boyd, Hamish W., M.D. *Introduction to Homeopathic Medicine*. New Canaan, CT: Keats Publishing, Inc., 1982.

The British Homeopathic Journal, Faculty of Homeopathy, London. Vol. LII, No. 4, 1963; Vol. LIV, No. 2, 1965; Vol. LIX, No. 1, 1970; Vol. LX, No. 4, 1971; Vol. LXXIII,, No. 3, 1984.

Capra, F. *The Turning Point*. London: Wildwood House, 1982.

Clark, John H., M.D. *A Dictionary of Practical Materia Medica* (Three Volumes). Saffron Walden, UK: The C. W. Daniel Co., Ltd.

Clarke, John H., M.D. *Clinical Repertory*. Saffron Walden, UK: The C. W. Daniel Co., Ltd.

Clark, John H., M.D. *The Prescriber*. Saffron Walden, UK: The C. W. Daniel Co., Ltd., 1987.

Cook, Trevor M., Ph.D. *The A-Z of Homeopathy*. Slough, UK: W. Foulsham & Co., Ltd., 1985.

Cook, Trevor M., M.D. *Samuel Hahnemann, Founder of Homeopathy*. St. Louis, MO: Formus, Inc., 1981. Wellingborough, UK: Thorsons Publishers, Ltd., 1981.

Cummings, Stephen and Ullman, Dana, M.P.H. *Everybody's Guide to Homeopathic Medicine*. Los Angeles, CA: Jeremy P. Tarcher, Inc., 1984.

Hahnemann, Samuel. *The Chronic Diseases, Their Peculiar Nature and Cure*. Calcutta, India: C. Ringer & Co., ND.

Hahnemann, Samuel. *Materia Medica Pura*, Vol. I, II. Translated by R. E. Dudgeon, M.D. New Delhi, India: B. Jain Publishers Ltd., ND.

Hahnemann, Samuel. *Organon of Medicine*. New Translation. Los Angeles, CA.: Jeremy P. Tarcher, Inc., 1984.

Hamlyn, Edward, M.D. *The Healing Art of Homeopathy*. New Canaan, CT: Keats Publishing, Inc., 1980.

Hering, Constantine, M.D. *Condensed Materia Medica*, 4th Edition. New Delhi, India: B. Jain Publishers Ltd., ND.

Kent, J. T., M.D. *Repertory of Homeopathic Materia Medica*, 6th U.S. Edition. New Delhi, India: B. Jain Publishers, Ltd., ND.

Pratt, Noel, M.D. *Homeopathic Prescribing.* New Canaan, CT: Keats Publishing, Inc., 1980.

Schauenberg, Paul and Paris, Ferdinand. *Guide to Medicinal Plants.* New Canaan, CT: Keats Publishing, Inc., 1977.

Scott, K. A., M.D., and McCourt, Linda A. *Homeopathy. The Potent Force of the Minimum Dose.* Wellingborough, UK: Thorsons Publishers, Ltd.

Smith, Trevor, M.D. *Homeopathic Medicine.* Wellingborough, UK: Thorsons Publishers, Ltd., 1983.

Speight, Phyllis. *Homeopathic Remedies for Women's Ailments.* Saffron Walden, UK: The C. W. Daniel Co., Ltd., 1985.

Tetau, Max, M.D. *Clinical Homeopathic Materia Medica and Biochemic Associations.* Paris, France: Maloine et Cie, 1986.

Tyler, Margaret L., M.D. *Homeopathic Drug Pictures.* Saffron Walden, UK: The C. W. Daniel Co., Ltd.

Wood, Clive. "Towards a Definition of Holism," *Holistic Medicine,* January/March, 1988.

INDEX

ABOUT THE AUTHOR

Dr. Trevor M. Cook, born in London, England, is known internationally for his contributions to homeopathy.

After studying at the University of London, he worked in research in the orthodox pharmaceutical industry, where he played a significant role in the development of several of the world's safest and most successful diuretic and antihypertensive drugs.

Dr. Cook was formerly Managing Director of Nelson's in London, where he held the Royal Warrant as manufacturer of homeopathic medicines to Queen Elizabeth II. Subsequently, he became President of the Dolisos Company, manufacturers of homeopathic medicines based in Las Vegas, Nevada.

He is a renowned lecturer in Europe and the United States, the author of many articles and papers on homeopathic topics, as well as the author of several books, including *Samuel Hahnemann, Founder of Homeopathy; The A to Z of Homeopathy*, and *A Beginner's Introduction to Homeopathy*. He has also taken part in numerous radio and TV programs to promote homeopathy worldwide.

Dr. Cook is President of the United Kingdom Homeopathic Medical Association and Principal of the Hahnemann College of Homeopathy, London.

He is Editor of *Homeopathy International*, a member of the Advisory Council of American Homeopathy, a Director of the Society of Ultramolecular Medicine and a member of the United States Pharmacopoeia Convention.